WEIGHT LOSS

Twenty Pounds
in
Ten Weeks

M.O.V.E. It to Lose It

Lt. Col. Bob Weinstein, USAR-Ret.

Take back control of your weight.
A no-nonsense, straightforward, weight loss and
weight management solution for all ages.

The Health Colonel Series™
www.TheHealthColonel.com

Weight Loss - Twenty Pounds in Ten Weeks - MOVE It to Lose It

By: Lt. Col. Bob Weinstein, USAR-Ret.
(Lt. Col. Joseph R. Weinstein, USAR-Ret.)
www.TheHealthColonel.com
757 SE 17th Street, #267
Fort Lauderdale, Florida 33316
954-636-5351

Copyright © 2009 Lt. Col. Joseph R. Weinstein, USAR-Ret.
All Rights Reserved.
ISBN-10: 0-9841783-0-9
EAN-13: 978-0-9841783-0-8
Published by The Health Colonel

The Health Colonel Series™

Printed in the United States

Library of Congress Control Number: 2009909978

Unless otherwise indicated, all scripture quotations are taken from the Holy Bible, New Living Translation, copyright © 1996. Used by permission of Tyndale House Publishers, Inc., Wheaton, Illinois 60189. All rights reserved.

Before beginning any exercise program, consult your physician. The author and publisher of this book and workout disclaim any liability, personal or professional, resulting from the misapplication of any of the training instructions described in this publication.

Cover Design by Emmy Shubert

What others are saying about this book:

This book offers just what is needed to stay fit and healthy and lose excess weight. When needed. No hype. No gimmicks.

- Dr. Ihor Pidhorecky, M.D., Surgical Oncologist

A straightforward, no-nonsense weight-loss book with a realistic ten week program that works.

- Dr. Jamie E. Marlowe, Ed.D., Combat Hospital Commander, former, Colonel, USAR-Ret.

Finally, an outstanding weight loss book that clearly covers exercise and eating that is realistic.

- Elizabeth Schy, RN, BSN, University of Miami-Humana Health Services Research Center

Read this before you start a weight loss and exercise program. It will get you focused on what matters most to lead a healthy lifestyle.

- Albert Miniaci, President of Paramount Companies, South Florida's industry-leader in vending for food service, amusements and coffee service

I have finally found my weight loss boot camp for life. This book offers just what is needed to stay fit and healthy and lose excess weight.

- LCDR Alan Starr, NSCC Regional Director, US Naval Sea Cadet Corps

WEIGHT LOSS

Twenty Pounds
in
Ten Weeks

M.O.V.E. It to Lose It

This book is dedicated to my wife Grit and my son David.

CONTENTS

YOUR M.O.V.E. TOOLBOX

About the Author

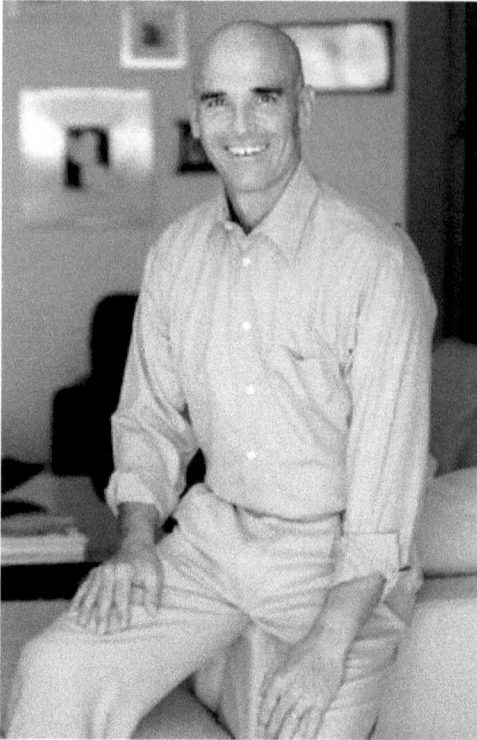

Lt. Col. Bob Weinstein, USAR-Ret.
www.TheHealthColonel.com

BIO

Born in Washington, D.C., Lt. Col. Bob Weinstein grew up in Virginia and spent 20 years in Berlin, Germany; he is retired from the United States Army Reserve as a Lieutenant Colonel with 30 years of service and spent about half that time as a senior military instructor with the Command & General Staff College.

He has been featured on radio and television, among others, on the History Channel and Fox Sports Net as well as in various publications such as the Washington Times, The Miami Herald and the Las Vegas Tribune.

His background is unique and diverse, including: military instructor, attorney, motivational speaker, wellness coach, certified corporate trainer, and certified personal trainer. He is fluent in German and English.

He is a popular motivational speaker at corporate events and banquets and conducts military-style workouts on Fort Lauderdale Beach utilizing strength, cardio, flexibility and agility training - both in personal training and group sessions.

He strongly believes in the importance of giving back to the community. Col. Weinstein volunteers his time for homeless and run-away kids at the Covenant House and also devotes time to training youth who are members of the US Naval Sea Cadets Corps , Team Spruance, Fort Lauderdale, Florida.

He is a member of the National Speakers Association and the American Council on Exercise.

He is the author of *Change Made Easy - Your Basic Training Orders to Excellent Physical and Mental Health.,* about personal development, fitness, exercise and health. Some of his previous clients as a guest speaker include: Sony, DHL, American Express, KPMG, AOL, IBM, AARP, SmithBarney, Green Bay Packers and Humana.

PREFACE

There is so much information and misinformation about weight loss on the market. Friends, acquaintances and clients have approached me many times with the comment and questions, "Bob, I'm confused. There's so much information and so many products and programs on the market offering weight loss solutions. Which ones are right? Which weight loss strategy has a lasting impact?" *Weight Loss - Twenty Pounds in Ten Weeks- M.O.V.E. It to Lose It,* answers these questions. The primary focus is and should be the long-term impact of everything you do, say and think. This book is designed to guide you on your healthy lifestyle journey and is results and solutions oriented without the hype or pie-in-the-sky promises often encountered.

You will not only find clear and simple guidance but will also get my "toolbox" to help you tackle weight loss found in this book under "YOUR M.O.V.E. TOOLBOX." You will also find some excellent free resources on the web, such as nutrition.gov and my web site TheHealthColonel.com.

Lt. Col. Bob Weinstein, USAR-Ret.
Fort Lauderdale, Florida

ACKNOWLEDGEMENTS

I want to sincerely thank all my Beach Boot Camp recruits and friends for the most rewarding time of my life and the great camaraderie. You are an enormous source of inspiration for me. Your inspiration is a significant contributor to this book.

I also thank my wife, Grit, for her love and moral support and her patience in allowing me to complete this book.

WARNING—DISCLAIMER

CHAPTER ONE

REAL WEIGHT LOSS STORIES FROM REAL PEOPLE JUST LIKE YOU

If you want to predict the future, take a close look at how you live. Everything you do, say and think has a long-term impact and will - to a great extent - determine your future.

Before we get into the nuts and bolts of weight loss, it is important that you put your weight loss and weight management journey into perspective. The best way to start is to be inspired by what others have accomplished. These weight loss stories are unedited so you will find out what Jeannette and Paul really think and how they have tackled weight loss. I know them both personally and they have been training with me for a while. Their stories have been an inspiration for me and many others.

HOW JEANNETTE LOST 67 POUNDS

FROM DRESS SIZE 18 TO 10

Jeannette has been attending my Beach Boot Camp group classes on Fort Lauderdale Beach for the past year and a half. She is 25 years old and did not really begin her weight loss journey until the age of 23. She is a 7th grade teacher and has a predominantly sedentary job. At 5'10" tall, her present weight is 173 lbs. She weighed 200 lbs in high school. Before she started her successful weight loss program at the age of 23, Jeannette weighed 240 lbs. She has lost 67 lbs of excess weight. She went from a size 18 to a 10-12.

Her BMI or Body Mass Index when she weighed 240 pounds was 34.4 which is obese on the BMI scale. Her present BMI weighing in at 173 pounds results in a BMI of 24.8 which puts her in the healthy range. Jeannette will share her own words how she took back control of her health and lifestyle.

Colonel Bob: What lessons have you learned on your weight loss journey?

Jeannette: Once I decided on losing weight I knew I would not be cured overnight. In fact, I am still not cured. I will always bear the challenges with food I have had since childhood. Once an addict, always an addict. It is the dedication to my program that will overcome the addiction to food.

It's also so important to hold myself accountable for the choices I make. It is vital to weigh myself everyday to monitor my progress or pitfalls. Recording my weight keeps me motivated to stay on track. In addition to weight, holding myself accountable for what I eat is just as important. My saying is, "If you bite it, write it." This allows me to be consistent with my food intake and make choices that will fill me up without bulking me up. This may include eating lots of veggies, switching to skim milk, and eating half of something when I may have previously eaten the entire thing.

Finally, finding support is probably the most important aspect in regards to my weight loss. Interacting with individuals who have the same goals, struggles, and determination keeps me going day after day even if I am tired of the entire ordeal. The feeling of showing up to Beach Boot Camp and seeing a group of smiling faces is encouragement I have not found anywhere else. My fellow bootcampers

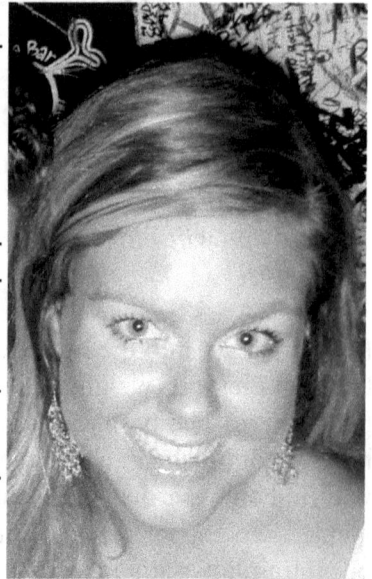

have the ability to turn sore legs into powerful ones and a feeling of defeat into triumph.

Colonel Bob: What were some of the phases of weight and eating habits you went through?

Jeannette: My entire life I have been overweight. This is due to bad learned habits from my parents who are also overweight. Eating well and exercise were not a part of our everyday life, but I was surely reminded on a daily basis that I was the fat girl. Seeing as how I was not raised with the correct tools to stay healthy I had to learn to eat healthy and control my weight on my own through exercise and diet.

My initial idea of weight loss was exercise = weight loss and I continued to eat as I pleased. This was effective for about 30 lbs of weight over a year's time frame. After the initial year, the weight started to pile back on. As it turns out, exercise is only half of the regimen.

After realizing I needed to change my eating habits as well I had no idea where to start as I had not been taught how to eat right. I started taking ideas from people - eating only protein, cutting down my portions, but nothing seemed to be effective. Soon after, a friend of mine introduced me to weight watchers. I was very skeptical but her results were fantastic so I gave it a whirl. Weight Watchers taught me what to eat and how much to eat. I learned to make my portions smaller, eat different foods, and pay attention to labels. The biggest gift weight watchers gave me is vegetables. Veggies are zero points! I can eat as much as I want and it will not pack on the pounds! A revelation! Being that I am a binge eater, binge eating on veggies allows me to work with my demons rather than against them, depriving myself as so many diets do. And not only can I eat as many as I'd like, but they are good for me! It's brilliant! Moreover, 6 months and 35 additional lbs later I realize nutrition and exercise go hand in hand for weight loss results.

Colonel Bob: What were your greatest challenges and how did you overcome them?

Jeannette: The challenges that come with weight loss are different for everybody and for me it is sticking to my program when I am around others who are not. It seems impossible to go out for a meal with friends and see the person next to me order a delicious, mouth-watering burger with tantalizing french fries. YUM! And I am sitting there with a plate of raw tuna and soy sauce, which is only 4 weight watchers points as opposed to 30. With experience I have learned that yes, the burger may be satisfying for that moment, but I will feel defeated for the next 3 days if I were to eat it. And believe me, I have been there, I have succumb to the fatty burger and sometimes a food hangover is worse than one brought on by a fifth of tequila. Overall, making good choices when out with friends ends up leaving me with a sense of pride and self worth.

Speaking of Tequila, another huge burden for me is when my friends, who are not on a program, want to go out and party at night. Not only is alcohol filled with calories, but it makes it impossible to get up for Beach Boot Camp on Saturday mornings. And I assure you, I've attempted hung over Beach Boot Camp and it's not pretty. Having to stand up to peer pressure can be one of the most challenging things in general, let alone when it's something that is super fun and I know I enjoy. I've simply learned to ask my friends to not even invite me on Friday nights and explain I will join them on a Saturday evening instead. This way everyone wins. For the most part, my friends support and encourage me to stick to my program, but there are always times when I am put to the test and getting past those hurdles are gratifying and make me stronger.

Colonel Bob: What keeps you on track?

Jeannette: Weight Watchers and Beach Boot Camp, of course are key to keeping me accountable when it comes to the everyday routine but it's the other, social aspects that keep me going.

I remember the first time I saw my parents after having lost a significant amount of the weight. My mother started crying! She was so proud of what I had accomplished. In fact, she has even started her own program. She is now eating better and has started swimming everyday. Seeing how much I influence others keeps me on track.

Every time I go the mall I seem to be able to buy smaller and smaller sizes. Recently I came out of a dressing room with a blue strapless dress on and it seemed the entire population of the fitting room had come to see how marvelous I looked in this dress. Ooooo hing and aaaahing at the glorious fit. I felt like a movie star. Having complete strangers tell me how great I look keeps me on track. For most of my life I was never popular with the opposite sex. I was not kissed until the age of 16 and not again until 18. As it turns out, guys do not want a fat girlfriend. This was always something that really bothered me and I had just accepted as fact. These days, I can't keep the guys at bay. My phone and email are filled with possible suitors who want ME, THE FAT GIRL, to be their girl-friend. All I have to say is the ball being in my court is what keeps me on track.

Colonel Bob: What is your weight history starting from high school?

Jeannette: All of high school I weighed more than 200 lbs and was always a size 16. I never attended school dances or functions as I was so ashamed and embarrassed about the way I looked. I never felt good enough or deserving enough because I was fat. Once I got to college I dropped some weight, although I don't know how much. Between the terrible dorm food and having to walk to class I slimmed down quite a bit. This helped me gain access to fun social things, like a sorority, although my weight loss was short lived. Apparently binge drinking and pizza will not keep the pounds off. And let me tell you, not being able to fit into the sorority shirts provided by the sorority is not good for sisterhood morale. By the time I graduated college I was 240 lbs and not feeling good about myself. It was a good thing jeans and hoodies were acceptable attire for college life. It really became a problem when at 240 lbs I had to start looking for a job and start buying "professional clothes." I remember when I bought my first suit. It was a suit skirt ensemble and the skirt had to have the elastic in the back and came from the women's department of Macy's. I cried and cried and cried - it was humiliating. Now at 173 I will put on that suit and stare in awe as to how much I've accomplished.

Colonel Bob: What changes have you made in your eating habits?

Jeannette: Previous to starting weight watchers I had no prob-lem eating very large meals 3 times a day. This may include fast food, eating out at restaurants or just eating the wrong foods at home.

A personal favorite being pizza roles - yum! Currently, I eat about six 200 to 300 calorie meals a day. This keeps me satisfied all day long. I still go out to dinner - I just order different food. A restaurant favorite of mine is rare tuna. It's something I would never make at home and it's extremely low in calories. White fish is a great restaurant treat as well. At home I eat mainly veggies and lean meats. And I can still have pizza - I just make my own on English muffins with fat free cheese. Its still delicious and it keeps me within my daily calorie range. I would like to say that my eating didn't have to change all that much, but in fact it did. It was all about educating myself about where I could cut calorie corners and what good alternatives to my favorite foods might be. At first it was challenging, but these days it seems effortless.

Colonel Bob: Did you use a support system or was someone else there to support and encourage you?

Jeannette: I had no trouble finding great motivators during my weight loss journey. Beach Boot Camp has been indispensable to me through this process. The support that comes with the group is unique and second to none. One thing in particular that means a lot to me in the way of Beach Boot Camp is at the end of every session, Col. Bob joins the "troops" together and gives a final motivational quote. During this time, I breathe deep, allowing the ocean air to fill my lungs and simply take a minute to be proud of myself for effort and the accomplishment. Bob reminds us daily that we are the few, we are the 1% and that is something I take to heart.

Additionally, the friends I have made there will be lifelong. We all share one thing in common - we want to maintain a healthy lifestyle. That in itself is something to cherish. Outside of bootcamp I have a dear friend named Kat. She introduced me to weight watchers and so many activities I would have never done on my own - biking, running, kayaking, and swimming. This network of people I have in my life put forth energy, focus, and determination that are totally contagious.

Even outside of my close relationships it is easy to find support. Everywhere I go I am sure to work into the conversation that I am on a program. For example, I was at a drug store yesterday and at the checkout the clerk asked if I would like to buy M&Ms as they were buy-one-get-one-free. I politely and graciously said, "No thank you. I am on weight watchers and those do not go well with my points system." Upon me saying that her face lit up. She asked me dozens of questions and even offered me her own story of her battles. People, in general, want to be a support system and want support. Not only was she supporting me by listening and engaging in conversation, but I may have left her with a twinge more motivation for her goals as well. Situations like this occur almost daily for me - it's about being open and honest with others about my struggles and my ultimate goal.

Colonel Bob: How do you see your health over the next five, ten and twenty years and how can you impact on your health over the long-term?

Jeannette: I'm hooked! I know I will be healthy for the rest of my life. I will never reach a point in my weight loss and say, "OK, I reached my goal, I am finished." Fitness and nutrition will always take a front seat in my life.

A huge example that is pertinent to my current life is dating. When I initially go on a date with someone the first things I inquire about are their personal habits. How much do they exercise, what sort of exercise they partake in, what is their diet like. These things are so important to me that I would not consider dating someone who did not have the same values I have regarding health. I am looking for a partner who wants to go for bike rides as opposed to a movie, go for a run as opposed to the bar. I refuse to end up with someone who may sabotage what I've worked so hard for. And if he can't hack Beach Boot Camp, then forget it!

Looking farther down the road, my children will grow up in a healthy home where nutrition and exercise are a way of life and something to be proud of. A life without being healthy is not a life at all - it's simply a means to death. I refuse to die as a result of self destruction.

Colonel Bob: Have you or do you have set-backs and how do you or have you overcome them?

Jeannette: I have set-backs all of the time! It comes with the territory. For me, it's about looking at the big picture. My biggest problem is that when I lose 10 lbs or so I seem to plateau for long periods of time. These are very frustrating, but I just have to remind myself that this is a part of my journey and they will pass. I also look at ways I can alter or improve my lifestyle to move past the halt in progress. This may mean stepping up the pace in Beach Boot Camp or analyzing what I'm eating in addition to how much I'm eating. It seems to be a matter of stepping back and taking in the overall picture of what I may need to do differently.

HOW PAUL LOST 40 POUNDS

Paul Kalil has been attending my Beach Boot Camp training on Fort Lauderdale Beach for fifteen months. He is 39 years old and has been overweight since childhood. At 5'8", Paul weighed approximately 240 pounds in high school, but lost 80 pounds in his senior year by moderating his calorie intake and exercising daily. Paul's weight fluctuated in the following years while he attended college, but he remained relatively fit and active and enjoyed running.. However, during law school and the ensuing years, Paul slipped into a sedentary lifestyle and gained significant weight. When he started the Beach Boot Camp program, he weighed in excess of 270 pounds. After nine months of training, he had lost over 40 pounds and completed his first half-marathon. Paul continues to struggle with his weight, but regular exercise and mindful nutrition keep him on the right path. He looks forward to many half-marathons in his future.

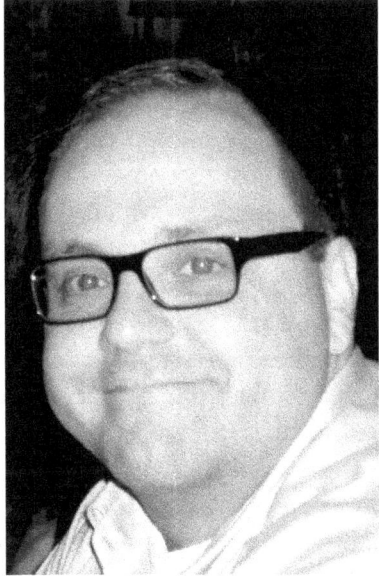

Colonel Bob: What lessons have you learned on your weight loss journey.

Paul: There is an exercise program for everyone. I never thought I would ever get involved with a fitness class. But I learned that exercise can double as entertainment if you choose the right activity for you, be it a class, a sport, or your own program.

I don't exercise just because I want to lose weight. I find activities that I really enjoy doing just for the sake of doing them. Through those activities, I have made friends, faced challenges and accomplished things I never imagined I could. The weight loss is almost an afterthought.

Colonel Bob: What were some of the phases of weight and eating habits you went through?

Paul: My weight fluctuations have always coincided with personal changes. I tend to eat less when I am stressed or distracted. I eat considerably more when I am inactive or bored.

I am addicted to carbs, especially sweets, but I find that I crave sweets less when I exercise regularly. I don't know if this is physiological or psychological, but it definitely is so.

My most recent weight loss has coincided with some significant lifestyle changes which have been both positive and negative, and have resulted in changes in diet and routine. Overall I have tried to stick to a reduced calorie, low sugar diet, and maintain my regular exercise routine. But I have fallen off the wagon from time to time and given in to cravings, or missed workouts here and there. Change is inevitable and nothing is forever. That includes good and bad habits, too.

Colonel Bob: What keeps you on track?

Paul: The people who travel with me, for the most part. I will admit that my motivation often comes from external sources, and not always from within.

Colonel Bob: What is your weight history starting from high school?

Paul: I have been overweight since I can remember. By my senior year of high school, I was 240 lbs. I lost 80 pounds that year by simply eating less and exercising moderately each day (brisk walking for an hour or so). My waist size went from 44 to 36 inches.

My weight fluctuated through college, and eventually I put about 40 lbs. back on.

After college I started running. I was relatively fit, and lost some weight, but I was still pretty heavy. I never weighed myself, but my blood pressure was quite low and my Resting Heart Rate was around 54.

Law school was the killer. All I did was study, commute and eat, for three years. By the time I graduated, I was back at 240 lbs., or more. For the next ten years, I continued to gain weight. When I started Beach Boot Camp I was over 270 lbs. (my scale maxed out at 270). Since starting Beach Boot Camp in May, 2008, I have lost over 40 lbs. I'm not sure exactly how much because my scale was maxed out when I started. I have gained about 12 pounds back in the last couple months, but I am now on the downward trend again.

Colonel Bob: What changes have you made in your eating habits?

Paul: I think my biggest change has been the reduction of sugar intake. Much fewer sweets, no more sugary cereals, and I look out for hidden sugar in other foods that appear to be healthy. I eat fruit in moderation, always mindful of the sugar.

No white bread. Ever. I do not keep bread at home anymore. But I still buy the occasional wheat bagel or sandwich on decent bread. Pasta is an occasional indulgence rather than a staple.

I have also eliminated most dairy products from my diet, especially cheese, which had been a big source of excess calories and fat/cholesterol.

Colonel Bob: Did you use a support system or was someone else there to support and encourage you?

Paul: Of course, I have had a lot of support from friends and co-workers who have noticed my weight loss and improved fitness. But the greatest encouragement has come from my fellow "Troops" at Beach Boot Camp. It is one of the few places where it seems that nobody wants someone else to fail. That has been crucial to my success.

Colonel Bob: How do you see your health over the next five, ten and twenty years and how can you impact on your health over the long-term?

Paul: At 39, I am already feeling the effects of a largely sedentary lifestyle and decades of bad habits. I have greatly improved my health in the last year, and barring some catastrophic illness or injury, I foresee continued improvements in health and fitness for the years to come. I can't control my genes, stop myself from aging, or change my past behavior, but I am confident that I can reduce my health risks and improve my quality of life staying active and maintaining responsible habits. But I know it will always be a struggle.

Colonel Bob: Have you or do you have set-backs and how do you or have you overcome them?

Paul: I have had some injuries from trying to do too much, too fast. Injuries are not only physically uncomfortable, the pain damages your confidence and leads you to question whether you can continue exercising. With training and weight loss come greater strength and better health. But there are times when you have to back off a little so you don't get hurt. When injuries happen (and they will happen) I try to keep things in perspective. The pain may be great, but the injuries aren't usually serious. The pain will go away, and I will be back to working out soon enough. When faced with any kind of adversity, I always try to remember: "This too shall pass."

I have also "fallen off the wagon" from time to time and indulged in bad food and laziness. When this happens, I accept it for what it is: a setback in my road to better health and fitness. I try not to get too down on myself when I do this. I see it as part of the process. It doesn't mean I have to continue down a bad path, it just means I need to set things right again. And I can set things right again.

CHAPTER TWO

The M.O.V.E. Weight Loss and Fitness Program

"An object at rest tends to stay at rest and an object in motion tends to stay in motion." - Sir Isaac Newton

We all need a little push or kick-start to get things going. The four month M.O.V.E.™ fitness and weight loss program is designed to create momentum in achieving your worthy goals of weight loss and/or improving on your fitness and health. *"An object at rest tends to stay at rest and an object in motion tends to stay in motion."* Those are the words of Isaac Newton addressing the First Law of Physics. You are the object he's talking about being in motion or at rest, whichever the case may be. If you are mostly leading a sedentary lifestyle – well, you are that object at rest that tends to stay at rest, which explains why it is so difficult to get some motion going. If you are that object in motion, your tendency is predetermined by the law of physics; your tendency is to remain in motion. My objective is to get that object (you) at rest to move, so that that object (you) stays in motion and on the M.O.V.E.™ The *ten week workout plan* which you'll find as a part of *Your M.O.V.E. Toolbox* is designed to give you a workout routine you can take care without the necessity of a gym.

M.O.V.E. ™ stands for:

> **M** AXIMIZE your results.
> **O** VERCOME your weaknesses and bad habits.
> **V** ICTORY. Achieve victory through lifestyle change empowerment.
> **E** NERGIZE. Become energized to accomplish all your worthy goals.

The Problem:

Extra Pounds, sedentary lifestyle, bad eating habits

- Are you looking to fit into that special dress? I'm talkin' about the ladies here -- or need I mention that?
- Are you looking to reverse the signs of aging?
- Are you having problems getting rid of that excess weight?
- Do you just want to look great in that new bikini?
- Are you ready to get that toned and firm body you have always wanted?
- Are you out of shape and getting more so?
- Don't know how to break those bad eating habits?
- Don't have time to exercise?
- Are you seeking to simply improve your fitness level?
- Are you looking to improve your health?

The Solution:

Your Own Fitness and Weight-loss M.O.V.E.™ Program

You can organize the M.O.V.E. program as an integral part of your fitness boot camp team or cell or at your gym, or you can just pair up using a buddy system. Some of the assessments may be beyond your expertise or beyond the expertise of your team members. That's okay. Check with your local gym, club or wellness coordinator to help you with some of them assessments, if necessary.

The M.O.V.E.™ Program includes:

- **Weight-Loss Goals** Established – You should not lose more than one to two pounds per week.
- **Eating Habits Assessed** – Perform a self-assessment or have a team member help you and apply the basics as set forth in this book on eating for performance and energy.
- **Eating Issues Identified** – The basic issues are either quantity and/or quality of food.
- **Eating and Fitness Action Plan** – Create a plan of exercise three to six days per week and put it in your calendar like a doctor's appointment you must attend or like a project assigned by your boss that you must complete.
- **Body Mass Index (BMI)** – Go to Diabetes.org of the American Diabetes Association to calculate your BMI online every four weeks. You'll find excellent tips for eating and exercise plans at Diabetes.org whether you have diabetes or not.
- **Body Measurements** taken every four weeks – Use a tailor's tape measure to take body measurements.
- **Fitness Test** every four weeks (Total of five fitness tests including initial testing).
- **Fitness Goals** established every four weeks – Based on your fitness tests.
- **Digital Photos** taken for before-and-after photos – Smile as you get into shape!
- **Ten Week Workout Plan** - Designed to help you successfully accomplish up to twenty pounds of weight loss in ten weeks. The ten week workout plan is a part of your *M.O.V.E. Toolbox.*
- **M.O.V.E. Toolbox** - The M.O.V.E. Toolbox will give you all the tools you need to accomplish your weight loss goals.

Benefits of M.O.V.E.

M.O.V.E. is the catalyst you need to make those lifestyle changes that will encompass all those areas of your life that are truly important to you. Feel and visualize the new you with the following benefits:

- Healthy weight and size.
- Sleep better at night.
- More brain power due to reduced stress.
- More energy to keep going.
- Master life planning skills to keep on track with what is best for your happiness.
- Heightened level of awareness about how to lead a healthy life.
- All the structure you need in the *M.O.V.E. Toolbox* to complete your task to lose and manage your weight.

We have a health pollution crisis going on in America. We are polluting our health by how we live.

CHAPTER THREE

Six Keys to Weight Loss

It has nothing to do with eating or exercise and has everything to do with how you think.

Since over-consumption of food combined with lack of physical activity have resulted in high numbers of Americans of all ages to be overweight, it is essential that I unlock the door to long-term weight-loss. I have identified six foundational keys to permanent weight-loss and management.

Six Keys to Weight Loss

#1 – No more excuses
#2 – Talk to win
#3 – Think to win
#4 – Eat to win
#5 – Like how you look
#6 – Move

These weight-loss laws leave the realm of the quick-fix society and will successfully lead to long-term weight-loss and weight management.

We all need a little body fat, so don't go trying to lose body fat till you're skin and bones and can't find anything to pinch. Washboard abs visible to the point of no fat may be unhealthy and may cause your immune system to suffer, making you susceptible to disease and illness.

OVERWEIGHT AND OBESITY EPIDEMIC IN AMERICA:

- According to a study by the Centers for Disease Control, Americans are consuming more calories, on average, than they were 30 years ago—200 to 300 calories a day more. That's 73,000 to 109,500 calories per year. 3,500 calories equal one pound of fat. If these are excess calories, that translates to 21 to 31 pounds of fat in one year!
- An estimated 300,000 premature deaths and more than $90 billion in healthcare costs can be attributed to inactivity and obesity.
- 50% of Americans are overweight, 33% are obese and as many as 40% of women and 25% of men are trying to lose weight at any given time.
- Americans spend at least $30 billion a year on commercial weight-loss programs and products, and another $5 to $6 billion on fraudulent products.
- Being overweight is the second leading cause of preventable death in the US.

OVERWEIGHT AND OBESITY EPIDEMIC GOES GLOBAL

- Between half and two-thirds of men and women in 63 countries across five continents – not including the US – were overweight or obese in 2006.
- Canada and South Africa led in the percentage of overweight people with an average BMI of 29 among both men and women in Canada and 29 among South African women.
- In Northern Europe, men had an average BMI of 27 and women 26.
- In Southern Europe, the average BMI was 28.
- In Australia BMI was 28 for men and 27.5 for women.
- In Latin America the average BMI was just under 28.

A BMI of 25 is deemed overweight and greater than 30 is obese.

Source: The International Day for the Evaluation of Obesity (IDEA) study.

BMI OR BODY MASS INDEX VALUES

- Underweight: Below 18.5
- Healthy weight: 18.5 to 24.9
- Overweight: 25 to 29.9
- Obese: 30 or higher

Go to Diabetes.org, type in BMI calculator and then calculate your BMI.

SELF-DECEPTION AT WORK

90% of Americans know that most people are overweight, but only 40% think they are overweight, according to a phone survey of 2,000 adults conducted by the Pew Research Center.

BEWARE OF SELF-DENIAL

So a huge portion of the US population is on a diet or counting calories in one way or another. 90% of those who lose excess weight, however, gain it all back within twelve months. Why? Because of their self-talk -- or maybe I should say self-deceit.

"I'm not really overweight. I'll just lose a few pounds and that will be that." Or they say, "I'll start exercising when I lose that excess weight." What a paradox!

DIETING NEVER WORKS (LONG-TERM)

This self-denial is a fatal error and one that keeps people spending billions every year on those fake programs and products. The truth is, dieting by itself doesn't work. So let me make it clear that this chapter is really not just about weight-loss. It's about addressing the real issue: the quality of your lifestyle and how you really feel about yourself and others. How you design your life inevitably dictates the quality of your health. Every decision you make in your life has consequences, good or bad. I want to empower you to live the life that will make you truly happy and fulfilled.

I don't measure success in pounds or inches lost, or how strong you are, or how fast you can run, or how great you look.

HOW TO MEASURE WEIGHT LOSS SUCCESS:

- Reduced health risk factors
- Improvement in medical conditions
- Improved quality of life
- Improved psychological functioning
- Decreased reliance on medications
- Positive self-image
- Regular physical activity
- Healthy eating

Many of my clients make promises about what they will do, without any commitment to, or belief in, what they said. You've probably heard, or maybe even said, "Sure, I'll be there" to an invitation, and then simply didn't show up or called that day with a fabricated reason for not attending. Many people who say "I'm going to eat right and exercise regularly" or "I'm going to lose 20 pounds and keep it off" do the same thing—they just don't show up or follow through.

WEIGHT LOSS KEY #1 - NO MORE EXCUSES

What you say to yourself and others has a greater impact on your life than you could ever imagine. We are creatures of habit. All our habits, both negative and positive, make up our lifestyle - how we live, both in the workplace and at home. Truth, honesty and integrity impact the quality of your life, from eating to exercise to your relationships. This is a sober fact, and here's the reason. The more you do what is right in the course of your life, the more motivated and energized you become, to continue on this path and to take it to the next level. It becomes fun and it changes your way of thinking for the better.

Doing the right thing begets more of doing the right thing. You actually will have more energy to do so simply by doing so.

Living a life filled with culturally acceptable untruths is harmful to your health. OK, OK, I mean lies. But you and I know that when a fib is not serious, we tend to call it something less than a lie - an exaggeration, perhaps - or an excuse. Here are some examples:

"Suzy, did you do your homework last night?"
"Yes, Mom. I did it while watching TV."
Suzy didn't even crack a book. But she didn't totally lie; she did watch TV.

"Hey Sam, how big was that fish you caught the other day?"
"Oh, man, you should have seen it. It was at least a 30-pounder."
Yeah, right! One that weighed about 10 pounds!

"Marilyn, have you been going to the gym regularly like you promised?"
"Well, yes, I've been going."
Sure, she's been going, all right. Going right past it on her way to the donut shop.

You may think these are harmless examples. They are not. How we respond in so-called harmless situations is the precursor of our responses when it really does count. When we exaggerate or make excuses, we are building a habit of not telling the truth, and we are programming our own behavior so that it becomes more difficult to even tell the truth. If we continue to follow this path, we eventually end up redefining "truth," so that the truth or doing the right thing or following through with worthy goals, such as changing eating habits, losing weight or getting in shape, will lose its meaning.

THE PARADOX OF EXCUSES

We become experts in creating excuses for why we can't do what we recognize to be important. Boy, does that sound like a paradox! Imagine that. Finding and creating excuses for not doing what you have recognized to be important in your life. Just the other day, I had a conversation with a young lady. We'll call her Brenda. The conversation went like this: "Brenda, how important is your health to you, on a scale of 1 to 10, with 10 being most important?"

Brenda responded without hesitation, "My health is one of the most important things in my life. I give it 10 points."

BRENDA'S PARADOX

"Well, Brenda," I asked, "How often do you exercise each week?" She answered reluctantly, "I don't really have the time to exercise."

"Wait a minute," I said. "Let me get this straight. You just told me that your health is one of the most important things in your life, but your actions don't correspond. Explain that to me." She could not.

So what does Brenda need to do? Her words and thoughts on the importance of health don't match her actions. You see, she has made it acceptable to herself to *understand* how important her health is. Not one bit more. She sees that as enough. No action. No follow-through. Just awareness. She even had a quick excuse to keep her from taking action. As Zig Ziglar, the famous motivational speaker and author, says, *"The chief cause of failure and unhappiness is trading what you want most for what you want now."* Brenda is trading her health for a little extra time now. What a paradox!

EXCUSES REQUIRE PRACTICE AND TRAINING

A lot of training goes into making excuses, and people spend time carefully thinking of plausible ones. There are even several websites devoted to the art of making excuses. I just looked at one called "The Mother of All Excuses." You can read or submit excuses for not going to work, skipping school, speeding, running a red light, having an accident, breaking dates, missing church, and more.

Some other excuse-generating websites are The Random Excuse Generator, IShouldBeWorking.com and Sick day Excuse Generator. Here are some of the excuses I found:

EXERCISE EXCUSES:

- My workout clothes don't match.
- My cat's depressed.
- It's a bad hair day.
- I don't have time to exercise.
- I didn't shave my legs.
- Somebody was using my treadmill.
- I'm too old.
- We're all going to die anyway.

EATING EXCUSES:

- Eating right costs too much.
- I can't fit in the recommended five daily servings of fruits and vegetables.
- I don't have time to eat right.
- My sweet tooth rules, so I can't eat well.
- I enjoy fast food too much to eat right.
- It doesn't matter that I have a lousy diet, because I take a vitamin pill.
- I eat too much to ever be able to eat right.
- Other people in my household eat poorly, so I do, too.
- We're all going to die anyway

TAKE CHARGE

No more excuses means doing what you say you are going to do and following through with the right thing. It's about personal account-ability. Excuses are a practiced form of giving up control to external circumstances or people. *Taking charge of your life means focusing on what you can do - possibilities talk. Excuses are impossibilities talk.* If you have recognized that weight management, healthy eating and regular exercise are priorities for you, but you practice *impossibilities talk* by programming yourself through excuses, you have made it impossible to succeed in this area. You have created a barrier or wall preventing positive change.

Have the courage to take that positive first step in the direction you have recognized is best for you. Once you have realized what is really important for your life in the long term and you are totally convinced that it is the right thing, pursue it like your life depended on it. Because it does. Eliminate all excuses.

BE PATIENT AND CONSISTENT

Embarking on a life of good habits doesn't have to be done in giant steps. Take it one small step at a time. Be kind to yourself and enjoy the journey. Allow for gradual change in the right direction for your life. Have enough patience to let time take its course. Any change in your diet or lifestyle that improves your personal health, however small, is a step in the right direction.

YOUR ACTION PLAN

WEIGHT LOSS KEY #1 – NO MORE EXCUSES

CONTINUE TO DO THIS

Write down and take action on one thing you will continue to do and talk about that calls for personal responsibility in what you say (Examples: Planning and accomplishing exercise every week, reducing or controlling portion sizes during all meals).

IMPROVE THIS

Write down and take action on one thing you say that you don't always follow through on, something that needs improvement because you have recognized that it is important for you (Examples: eating lots of fruits and vegetables, reducing bread consumption, cutting out sweets).

STOP DOING THIS

Finally, write down and take action on one excuse about your health that you will stop using and the positive, empowering statement you will replace it with. For instance, instead of "I'm too tired" or "I'm too busy" or "It's a bad hair day," use Possibilities Talk: "I'll make the time and schedule exercise four to six times a week to be a part of my life, and I will follow through." Put it in your weekly calendar.

WEIGHT LOSS KEY #2 - TALK TO WIN

Discouraging and disempowering talk and self-talk will drain you of the positive emotions you need to accomplish life's many tasks, excel at work and nurture relationships.

What you say to others and yourself plays a key role in how successful you will be in bringing about positive change in your life. Every word of praise or kindness to others, or to yourself, actually programs you in a very positive and beneficial way.

You know eating properly and exercising are both positive. Right? How do you talk about these topics? Are you making empowering statements or disempowering ones? Are your thoughts focused on the positive or are they burdened by negative undertones? Remember that negativity is more than just the words you say!

There are emotions behind everything we say. Emotional energy is a primary source of life energy. Discouraging and disempowering talk will drain you of the positive emotions you need to accomplish life's many tasks, excel at work and nurture relationships. "Talk to win" refers to nonverbal communication as well. Walk, talk, stand and act with confidence. It will support you emotionally in the accomplishment of your worthy goals.

90% of those who lose excess weight, gain it all back within twelve months. Why? Because of their self-talk, or maybe I should say self-deceit. Let's examine the language we use about eating and exercise with Give-up vs. Take-charge talk.

GIVE-UP VERSUS TAKE-CHARGE TALK

Give-up: Should I have it?
Take-charge: Do I need it? Do I want it?

Give-up: I'll be successful once I lose those twenty pounds.
Take-charge: I am successful. I am listing and putting in my calendar what I need to do and I am implementing my goals now.

Give-up: I want it all or nothing.
Take-charge: I will take a gradual and long-term approach, one step at a time. I will do what I can do and never give up, because the cause is worthy.

Give-up: I eat when I'm stressed.
Take-charge: I eat when I'm hungry.

Give-up: I can only feel good about myself if I lose that weight.
Take-charge: I accept and like myself as I am with or without excess weight.

Give-up: Exercise means "no pain, no gain."
Take-charge: I like energetic daily living. It's fun! It's nature's Viagra. It gives me more energy.

Give-up: The diet is in control. I have no choice.
Take-charge: I am in charge. I decide what and when to eat.

Give-up: Food is the enemy. I have to deprive myself and use willpower.
Take-charge: Food is my friend and is there for my enjoyment. I decide what I eat.

Give-up: I don't have time to exercise.
Take-charge: Exercise gives me energy so I can use my time more productively. Exercise belongs in my calendar, whether it's for 10, 20, 30 or 60 minutes. It all adds up.

YOUR ACTION PLAN

Weight-loss Key #2 – Talk To Win

Transform something that you say that sounds like "I give up" and convert it to "I take charge." That's an order! Commit to never using that give-up-responsibility-talk again and to sticking with your new take-charge-talk.

WEIGHT-LOSS KEY #3 -THINK TO WIN

Your thoughts and emotions play a key role in all aspects of your health, not just in losing weight. Your mind can heal by mobilizing your body's natural healing powers. You have to watch how you program your thoughts and where your thoughts dwell. Where your thoughts predominantly dwell is the difference between winning and losing. This is not snake oil. If you give up hope, the battle is lost without ever firing a shot.

PLEASURE/PAIN PRINCIPLE

This step may be trickier than you think. Your subconscious is constantly trying to trick you. Even though you may completely understand that a certain behavior is the right thing to do, your subconscious starts working to get you back to where you were, where you were comfortable. This is called the pleasure/pain principle. Your subconscious is resistant to change because change is usually associated with pain. This is what was happening with Brenda when she rated her health as a 10 and yet did not devote the necessary time.

Bad habits are the primary cause of poor health. Our mission is to replace these bad habits with healthy ones. By replacing the bad habits with good ones, you will actually enjoy the new habits as well

FOCUS ON THE POSITIVE

Think positive thoughts about yourself and what is best for your health. Create a new association of pleasure when thinking about those positive changes in your exercise and eating habits, and treat yourself with kindness—like you would treat your best friend. This will replace the tendency to dwell on negative thoughts about weight-loss.

TREAT YOUR WEIGHT-LOSS GOAL LIKE YOU'VE ALREADY ACHIEVED IT.

SEE IT!

FEEL IT!

HEAR IT!

TASTE IT!

EMBRACE IT!

See, hear and feel the world around you. Visualize how you want to be NOW. Feel the benefits and rewards NOW. Listen to the sounds that are associated with it NOW. You can do this. This potential is in you. Tap into it and imagine it NOW, to experience the positive change. Knock that "T" off of "CAN'T." If you say you can't, you can't. If you say you can, you can. Bring back those enormous visualization capabilities you had as a child.

TAKE INVENTORY OF YOUR THOUGHTS

Here's a self-evaluation that's easy to do and can be fun and challenging while exploring your potential. Follow your thoughts for one or two days. List your negative and positive thoughts. Listen very carefully, because we are masters at tricking ourselves. Practice awareness of what you're thinking about yourself and others.

Are you overly critical? Overly negative? Compassionate? Allowing wisdom to rule? Always asking yourself how you would like to be treated, especially if you're not treating someone else that way? Use the Golden Rule and work on making those corrections every day. Don't kick yourself. Just say to yourself, "I'll do it better next time." Wherever you identify a predominant focus on negativity and complaining, turn it around. Think solutions- oriented thoughts and negativity and complaining will cease. Better yet, you will feel better and accomplish more, too.

TREAT YOURSELF LIKE YOU WOULD A BEST FRIEND

From now on, look at yourself and say nice things. Imagine the best way of treating someone special in your life and think such thoughts about *you*. Smile and say, "Hey, I like myself. I have made a mistake, but I can learn from it and do better next time. I like to enjoy life. I like to relax. I like to be good to myself. I'm worth it." That's how you would treat a friend. Be very *kind* to *you*. This will cause you to be kind to others. You will then reap more kindness in your life. Learn to forgive yourself and others and learn to move on.

As the famous motivator, Brian Tracy, says, *"Set peace of mind as your highest goal and organize your entire life around it."* Think carefully about the situations, people and settings that give you peace of mind. Learn from them. Start taking a gradual approach, one step at a time. Does it give you peace of mind to know that you are doing things and focusing on values that enhance your health? Of course!

YOUR ACTION PLAN

WEIGHT-LOSS KEY #3 – THINK TO WIN

Take charge of your thoughts and your mind. You decide where they wander and where they dwell. Your thoughts are to focus on positive things that benefit you and others. Doing so takes your eyes off of the obstacles and keeps you on track. If you fall and if you wander off track, get up, dust yourself off and continue to march.

GO THROUGH, OVER AND AROUND ALL OBSTACLES

Focus on what you want to accomplish and not on the obstacles, and you will begin to have the feeling that there are no obstacles. That's because you now have your sights on your worthy goals. If there's a wall there, you will simply approach it and immediately go to work on a way over, through or around it.

Norman Vincent Peale sums this step up best: "A positive thinker does not refuse to recognize the negative; he [or she] refuses to dwell on it. Positive thinking is a form of thought which habitually looks for the best results from the worst conditions." In other words, dwell on positive thoughts even under negative circumstances. Dwelling on positive thoughts means focusing on what you want to accomplish, not those bumps in the road, those fires to deal with or mountains to climb. There are no quick fixes for weight-loss or weight management or life. Only your determination to make positive changes can make positive changes.

These first three laws to permanent weight-loss - #1 No More Excuses, #2 Talk to Win, #3 Think to Win - make up about 80% of your success, so concentrate on them. They are performance enhancers and success multipliers. The rest of the keys are only responsible for about 20% of your success, and that is because the first three secrets will drive your success (or failure).

WEIGHT LOSS KEY #4 - EAT TO WIN

Have you ever wondered why, for so many people - especially anyone older than 30 in the U.S. - weight gain seems to be a fact of life? It's because the human body is way too efficient. It doesn't take much energy to maintain the human body at rest. And, when exercising, the human body is amazingly efficient when it comes to turning food into motion.

1,800 CALORIES TO STAY ALIVE

Those 1,800 calories are used to do everything you need to stay alive:

- They keep your heart beating and lungs breathing.
- They keep your internal organs operating properly.
- They keep your brain running.
- They keep your body warm.

312 MILES ON A GALLON OF GAS

If you could drink gas and digest it, you would get 312 miles on a gallon of gas. At $2.90 per gallon that would be about $0.01 per mile. I don't think I need to mention this but I will anyway. Don't drink gas. It will kill you!

In motion, the human body uses energy very efficiently. For example, a person running a marathon—which is 26 miles, or 42 km—burns only about 2,600 calories. In other words, you burn only about 100 calories per mile when you're running. Still, the body is designed to be used. If you don't exercise, your muscles will deteriorate, your arteries could clog, and your heart will have a harder time

pumping enough oxygen to the body. In short, you'll age and die faster.

Did you know that if we could drink gas and the body could actually process it as food, you would get about 912 MPG while bicycling? Now, that's great gas mileage! A gallon of gas has 31,000 calories.

If you have been dieting, you may be out of touch with your body and its signals for hunger and fullness. To get back in touch, you can do several things.

EAT REGULARLY

At least every three to six hours. Include breakfast, lunch and dinner . Add a snack if your body really signals the need. If you are physically hungry, do not fill up on water or coffee – eat something. Why? It's about getting back in touch with what your body says about hunger and responding to it. It takes three to six hours to digest a balanced breakfast, so you will be hungry by lunch time. If you eat these meals and stop eating when you're full, you will ultimately eat less at the evening meal and throughout the evening. Ignoring your natural hunger signals and under eating early in the day inevitably lead to overeating - even bingeing - later on. Eating regularly involves resetting your internal clock to a regular pattern of meals. Once you are in the habit of eating breakfast within an hour of getting up, you will soon start waking up hungry for the morning meal.

So what if you don't eat breakfast? About 50% of overweight people do not eat breakfast. Breakfast is the most important meal, so a nutritious breakfast should not be skipped.

What about more frequent meals, say, five to six times a day? Be careful with this one. It may lead you to eating more than you should, because you could eat only to not miss one of those six frequent meals. Eat when you are hungry and develop the habit of eating a nutritious breakfast. If you normally don't eat breakfast, ease into it by having just a little, such as half of a banana, and working your way up to a regular sized breakfast. You should eat at least three meals a day.

EAT BALANCED MEALS

The basic premise of any good diet is variety, moderation, and balance. Let's make this step really easy. Divide your plate into thirds: One third for protein (meat, seafood, poultry, and beans) and the other two thirds for vegetables, bread, potatoes and/or pastas.

"Well, instead of figuring out portions, I'm just going to get a really big or really small plate." If that helps you to adjust, that's great. Remember the focus. It's not about legal or illegal food. It's about getting back in touch with your body and responding to its real physical hunger and basic needs and what will satisfy you, while seeking out the most nutritious choices. A healthy lifestyle is one of both moderation and balance.

HIGH-OCTANE FOOD

So let's go back to dividing your plate into thirds and follow the **15/30/55 RULE**—15% protein, 30% fat and 55% carbohydrates. If a race car driver had to use food for his race car, this would be the formula for ultimate performance, as long as the ingredients over-whelmingly are unprocessed, unrefined, highly nutritious food. No race car driver is going to put low-octane fuel in his car. No human being should put low-octane food in his body. That will impact health and performance. This does not exclude once-a-week moderate amounts of sweets or desserts. More than once a week on a regular basis is too much.

PROTEIN DOES NOT JUST RUN AROUND ON TWO OR FOUR LEGS

We all have a tendency to only count the protein that comes from animal sources, and that includes dairy. We tend to disregard the protein that comes from plant sources, thereby eating too much protein. That is hard work for the kidneys and could indicate that you are either eating too much or you're not getting enough of the nutrient-rich plant products, such as fruits, vegetables, whole grains, beans and nuts.

Eat animal products no more than once a day while eating nutrient-rich, plant-based foods, and you will give your health a big boost. As a matter of fact, complete elimination of animal products while supplementing with calcium and Vitamin B-12 is extremely healthy.

15/30/55 RULE

How much food should you eat to follow the 15/30/55 guidelines? Now we're back to the topic of calories (and quantity), which doesn't necessarily mean more food. 200 calories of vegetables take up about the same amount of space as 1,000 calories of pasta! Your body will tell you how much to eat, if you "listen" carefully and closely. And if your body is still in the learning phase of "listening," a little old-fashioned, timeless, self-discipline will do the trick.

CHOOSE MEALS AND SNACKS THAT SATISFY

If you eat what you want, you will eat less in total. You need to eat enough to fill up—food that you like. But you also need to be careful to balance carbohydrates for energy—especially more complex carbs such as sweet potatoes, oatmeal or beans—with enough protein to keep you satisfied. This balance is what keeps you satisfied until it's time to eat again.

TAKE YOUR TIME

Effective eating takes time. You need to find out how good it feels to sit down to a meal pleasantly hungry and to take your time with it. You will end up satisfied and able to forget about eating between mealtimes. On the other hand, don't go telling yourself you're not going to eat a meal or healthy snack if you can't eat it slowly. That would be a fatal error. Do not skip a meal if you can avoid it. Gulp it down if you can keep it down and continue to work or do whatever you are doing.

GET ENOUGH FIBER

25 to 30 grams of fiber a day from unprocessed, close-to-nature food is a nutrient-rich diet. A fiber-rich diet helps your body deliver nutrients to its cells. If processed food and supplements are the sources of your fiber intake, you are probably not getting a sufficient amount of nutrients, which leads to an unhealthy diet. Does that mean you have to eat a can of beans a day? I think you and I know what could happen if you did that. No, eat more green and yellow-orange vegetables, citrus and yellow-orange fruits, and whole grains.

DRINK WATER

Water is one of the four basic nutrients the body needs. The other three are protein, carbohydrates and fats. Just about every process in your body depends on water. It is the most important detoxifier available to you. It helps clean you through your skin and kidneys, helps you look younger and, yes, helps you lose weight. Even mild dehydration will slow down your metabolism as much as 3%. The slower your metabolism is, the slower your weight-loss will be. You need to drink at least eight 8-ounce glasses a day. That's right. 64 ounces a day. Depending on the weather and the types of activities, you may need more. Not iced tea, not diet soft drinks, not powdered mixes, not fruit-flavored water in a bottle. Plain old water. Now quick. Go run and get a glass of water. I know this sounds really strict. If you feel the need to add some natural fruit flavor without the calories, by all means do so. Gradually back off of the flavoring to get used to drinking plain old H_2O again.

WHAT'S IN THAT CANTEEN, SOLDIER?

During a military training exercise many decades ago, I was stopped by a drill instructor who inspected my canteen to make sure I had water in it. He unscrewed the lid and performed a sniff test. Detecting a smell other than water – no, it wasn't whiskey or gin or any other alcoholic beverage! – he poured some of the contents onto the ground.

As he saw the bright red color of my "water," he barked at me, "That's not water!"
I quickly responded, "No, Sir!"
"What's that in your canteen, Soldier?" he shouted while I stood at attention.
"Kool-Aid, Sir!"
His barking was now getting louder, "Kool-Aid? You've got to be kidding me!"
"No, Sir! Kool-Aid!"
"That'll cost ya', Soldier! You're now officially promoted to KP duty for a week."

For those civilians who don't know what KP is, it stands for Kitchen Police and entails every imaginable kitchen duty necessary to service hundreds of troops, from mopping floors to washing dishes.

I thought I could get away with a little sweet beverage in my canteen. Red Kool-Aid was not the best choice, since my lips, gums and mouth were red. A dead give-away.

So, was my drill instructor right? Was it better to drink water without the added calories? You bet he was! One of the biggest and most consistent sources of additional daily calories is through the beverages that we regularly drink. The only exception I would make would be for the high performance athlete or for long workouts in heat and humidity.

TRAINING IN HEAT AND HUMIDITY

While training or working in heat and humidity, profuse sweating leads to electrolyte depletion. Electrolytes are substances that become ions in solution and acquire the capacity to conduct electricity. The balance of electrolytes in our bodies is essential for normal functioning of our cells and our organs. Common electrolytes are sodium, potassium, chloride, and bicarbonate.

The major electrolytes are:
- sodium (Na^+)
- potassium (K^+)
- chloride (Cl^-)
- calcium (Ca^{2+})
- magnesium (Mg^{2+})
- bicarbonate (HCO_3^-)
- phosphate (PO_4^{2-})
- sulfate (SO_4^{2-})

Electrolytes are important because they are what your cells (especially nerve, heart, muscle) use to maintain voltages across their cell membranes and to carry electrical impulses (nerve impulses, muscle contractions) across themselves and to other cells. Kidneys help keep the electrolyte concentrations balanced. During a heavy workout, especially in heat and high humidity, you lose electrolytes in your sweat, particularly sodium and potassium. These electrolytes must be replaced to keep the electrolyte concentrations of your body fluids constant. Many sports drinks have sodium chloride or potassium chloride added to them.

JUICES AND FLAVORED BEVERAGES

One level teaspoon of sugar has 16 calories and 4 grams of carbohydrate. One rounded teaspoon is actually 1-1/2 level tsps and 24 calories with 6 grams of carbohydrate. Now, let's take a look at how many teaspoons of sugar are actually in the following beverages.

Orange Juice, one 8-oz. glass, fresh pressed: 112 calories (Note: most containers have 2.5 servings, resulting in 280 total calories. 8 oz. has 21 grams of sugar or 5-¼ level teaspoons of sugar. If you buy and drink the container with 2.5 servings, you are then taking in 52.2 grams of sugar, or over 13 level teaspoons of sugar.

Gatorade, 8-oz serving, 50 calories, 14 grams of sugar which translates to over 3 level teaspoons of sugar. Ever see an 8-oz bottle of Gatorade? They're usually 16 or 24-oz containers.

Soft drink such as Coke or Pepsi, 12 oz, 155 calories, 40 grams of sugar which translates to 10 level teaspoons of sugar. Look at this! That 2.5-serving container of orange juice has more sugar than a 12-oz can of soda.

Smoothie, Banana Berry from Jamba Juice, Original size (719 grams), 518 calories, 107 grams of sugar or over 26 level teaspoons of sugar. Now, that's a sugar fix!

Starbucks Caramel Frappuccino® Light Blended Coffee, Grande (16 oz), 160 calories, 21 grams of sugar and 1.5 grams of fat.

Starbucks Caramel Frappuccino® Blended Coffee, Grande (16 oz), 380 calories, 48 grams of sugar and 15 grams of fat. **Starbucks Dulce de Leche Frappuccino® Blended Crème,** Grande (16 oz), 530 calories, 71 grams of sugar and 15 grams of fat (including 9 grams of saturated fat).

EAT GOOD FAT

Let's move on to another of the four nutrients the body needs, fat. A healthy diet includes fat, good fat. The secret to weight management is not avoiding fats or eating fats. It's understanding the difference between good and bad fat.

Fat from plant sources is better and healthier for you than fat from animal sources. If your fat intake is made up of saturated, hydrogenated and Trans fats, it may have a negative impact on your health. You may not feel ill. You may just feel tired or lethargic. No more than 10% of your diet should include saturated fat, which of course means that a little regular saturated fat will probably not harm you. But Trans fats, which can be found in canola oil, soy oil, corn oil, and anything called salad oil or vegetable oil, are very bad, because they are processed with high heat to make the oils stable for a longer shelf life. Read the labels carefully. New FDA standards require that the label includes information on Trans fats.

UNPROCESSED FAT FROM PLANTS IS GOOD

Focus on getting your fat from unprocessed plant sources, such as raw nuts or flax seeds that you can grind in the coffee grinder. Also, coconut, olive, peanut and sesame oils are examples of good fats as long as they are cold-pressed. Also eat lots of fatty fish, because it contains Omega-3, a fatty acid that the body can't produce on its own. Fatty fish include mackerel, lake trout, herring, sardines, salmon, and albacore tuna—even the canned, white-chunk kind.

Please be aware that there are issues with toxins in fish. Any predatory fish will generally have more poisons because it eats lots of other fish and therefore collects the toxins in its body. Non-predatory fish can also be a source of higher levels of poisons if they are farm-raised and fed fish parts as food.

You do have another excellent natural source of Omega-3 fatty acids. Omega-3's are also found in flax seeds. Just grind them up in a coffee grinder and use them for cooking, on cereals, and in salads. This is a great alternative for vegetarians and non-vegetarians. Good fats protect against aging, improve the immune system, balance hormone production, and improve brain function and vision.

SPICE IT UP

Herbs and spices are a concentrated source of antioxidants and other plant factors. And besides, they make some dishes taste better. Get creative with spices to make healthy, close-to-nature food taste very good. The eight basic spices are:

- Salt
- Pepper
- Onion
- Red pepper
- Basil
- Paprika
- Cumin
- Garlic

ARE YOU PREDATOR OR PREY?

Treat your trip to the grocery store like a hunt. You know that every hunt has prey and predator. So which are you when you grocery-shop?

If you sometimes feel like prey, you're not alone. Here's a sign I saw in the ice cream department of a grocery store: "1 to 12 servings, depending on how your day went." That sign is an attempt to make you the prey! Don't let it happen! Explore the options, read the labels, and carefully look for whole foods that are closer to nature, unprocessed. "Unprocessed" means food that has not been manipulated or has been minimally manipulated by man.

I never saw twinkies, white bread or pasta grow on a tree. Have you? It's processed food.

Which kind of oatmeal is processed? The instant kind or the stuff you have to cook on a stove? The kind you have to cook, of course. Which are processed, canned or frozen vegetables? Canned, of course. What about sandwich meats from the deli? Most of the sandwich meats are high in chemicals and salt and are highly processed and very unhealthy. What about foods labeled organic? Don't fall for it. Organic could be processed or natural.

The food-processing industry has managed to convince most of us that we are getting nutritional value from many processed foods, but it just isn't true. What we're actually getting is chronic malnutrition.

BE CAUTIOUS WHILE GROCERY SHOPPING

Be alert when grocery shopping. Be on the hunt. You will be surprised at the discoveries you will make, and you will raise your awareness about just what is healthier for your body and what to avoid. What to avoid is easy. Stay away from junk food and munchies—which are usually high in fat, sugar and/or salt. Eliminate, or at least greatly reduce, sugar. Replace diet beverages with water. Forget those fast-food joints even exist. When dining out, take charge of the dinner table, the server, and the menu, and you will eat healthier.

YOUR ACTION PLAN

WEIGHT LOSS KEY #4 – EAT TO WIN

EAT CLOSE-TO-NATURE

The less food is manipulated by man, the healthier it is. Eat predominantly plant-based foods, because that is where the vast majority of nutrients can be found that will help the body live disease-free, have more energy, fight off illness, and actually feel better.

15/30/55 RULE

Remember the rule of thumb: 15/30/55. Approx. 15% protein, 30% fat and 55% carbohydrates. Remember to count the plant-based protein. Also, test yourself for two to three typical days. Write down everything you eat and drink including all snacks, beverages and vitamin pills. Now calculate the calories and approximate the percentages of protein, fat and carbs. You may be surprised at the quantity (= calories) and percentages of protein, fat and carbs. Think about how you will adjust and, if necessary, make those changes and adjustments.

AVOID THOSE LOW-CARB OR HIGH PROTEIN DIETS

Stay away from those diets of low carbs or high protein or any of these other fancy ideas to get you away from healthy eating habits that are long-term.

BALANCE QUANTITY AND QUALITY

Remember that your primary eating issues are quantity and quality. Your mission is to keep an eye on both. Reduce the quantity, if necessary, and increase the quality of food you are eating.

WEIGHT LOSS KEY #5 - LIKE HOW YOU LOOK

Let's move on with our Offensive Weight-loss and Management Operations. No defensive posture here. Offensive means take the initiative and take charge of the battlefield. Secret #5 to reveal your own lifestyle based weight-loss program is to like how you look no matter how you look.

CAN YOU MORPH INTO A DIFFERENT BODY TYPE?

Did you know that there are three different body types? All of us fit into one of these types, or we may have elements of several. They are:

- **Endomorph** is a heavy body with a soft and rounded shape.
- **Mesomorph** is a well-developed, muscular body.
- **Ectomorph** is a long and lean body.

Bill Clinton, John Goodman, and Roseanne Barr are endomorphs. Arnold Schwarzenegger, Daryl Hannah, and Kevin Costner are mesomorphs. Mia Farrow, Anthony Perkins, and Fred Astaire are ectomorphs.

DOES IT MATTER WHAT BODY TYPE YOU ARE?

Which are you? It doesn't really matter. Whatever your body type is, you can't change it. What is important to remember is that regardless of your body type, you can be healthy by eating right and exercising regularly.

An important truth to remember for all body types is that regular exercise and healthy eating will make you look better and give you more energy.

If you look better and have more energy and you allow it to shine, others will notice, too. This is extremely important because of the unrealistic "ideal" body that is perpetrated in the media. I can assure you that there are people with these bodies who are not healthy. I also know people who have a little excess extra body fat who are very healthy because of the quality of food they eat and the active lifestyles they lead.

HERE'S WHAT YOU CAN CHANGE

What you can change is how you feel about how you look. Your feelings about your looks closely tie in with how you feel about yourself. Are you really going to begin to like yourself once you achieve that ideal weight and appearance? What if you never achieve it? Does that mean that you will not accept and like yourself as much? If your thoughts have led you to believe that you first must achieve that ideal weight before you can really be satisfied or like yourself, you are in for a rude awakening. You would not treat a friend like that, because you know the true worth of a friend is not their appearance or their state of health. You won't find happiness like that, and you will therefore probably have greater difficulty accomplishing some of your life goals because you will have robbed yourself of your greatest motivator. That's you!

YOUR ACTION PLAN

WEIGHT LOSS KEY #5 – LIKE HOW YOU LOOK

You are to like and respect yourself every single day! That means respectful thoughts and actions all the time. Never talk down to yourself or say demeaning things to yourself or to others about yourself. Treat yourself like you would a very best friend. Value who you are, and you will enhance your daily task performance, and your successful weight management will be within your reach. Now, there is a side benefit to this approach. You will have a lot more fun and enjoyment with life and you will enjoy being around YOU. There is another side benefit. Others will enjoy being around you much more and you will attract like-minded people into your life.

WEIGHT LOSS KEY #6 - MOVE!

The final secret to successful weight-loss and weight management requires you to move that body.

DEVELOP A PHILOSOPHY OF MOVEMENT

Develop a philosophy of movement in your life. Incorporate as much exercise and movement into your daily life as reasonably possible. Seek out activities-based things to do with your free time.

REGULAR MOVEMENT AND EXERCISE HAVE MANY BENEFITS

- ❑ Exercise helps control your weight because it helps burn calories.
- ❑ Exercise strengthens your body and makes it more fit and resilient.
- ❑ Exercise builds muscle, which will allow your body to burn even more calories at rest.
- ❑ Exercise strengthens your immune system.
- ❑ Exercise promotes healing and tissue regener -ation.
- ❑ Exercise promotes stress management.
- ❑ Exercise helps keep your heart healthy.
- ❑ Exercise promotes psychological wellness.

MOVEMENT PROMOTES FAT LOSS AND MUSCLE GAIN

Weight-loss without exercising will result in only 3/4-pound of fat loss and 1/4-pound of muscle loss for every pound lost. Weight-loss with an exercise program will result in 1 ¼-pounds of fat loss and a ¼-pound gain in muscle mass for every pound lost. This is based on a safe weight-loss program of 1 to 2 pounds per week.

EXERCISE STRENGTHENS YOUR IMMUNE SYSTEM

Exercise and movement actually promote the strengthening of your immune system. Your lymphatic system plays an important role in the strength of your immune system. The lymphatic system collaborates with white blood cells in lymph nodes to protect the body from being infected by cancer cells, fungi, viruses or bacteria. There is no pump – like the heart – to pump lymphatic fluid through the system, so exercise supports the movement of lymphatic fluid and the functioning of the lymphatic system. Conversely, a sedentary lifestyle may weaken your immune system.

Find a type or types of exercises that you enjoy and do it every day for a minimum of 30 minutes. It might be walking, running with your dog, dancing, riding a stationary bike while watching TV or reading, or even cutting the grass. All movement/exercise is cumulative. That means every 10, 15, 20, 30, 40 and 60 minute time period for exercise/movement adds up to a cumulative health benefit. Every minute spent watching TV will accumulate into hours, days, weeks, months and years of being sedentary.

Don't like to exercise? Tough! You are hereby ordered to like exercise. Spend every morning and evening in front of the mirror expressing your fondness of exercise and how you can hardly wait to move and exercise. This is not a joke.

Not liking exercise may kill you before your time or cause you to dome down with a disease or incapacitation that will not be fun.

TAKE THE STAIRS

Instead of taking the elevator, take the stairs. Park farther away from stores when you go to the mall. Put a set of weights at your desk and use them three or four times during the day as you think or talk on the phone. Walk whenever you can, not whenever you have to. Walking is an ideal and natural form of exercise. It's free, it's easy, and it's convenient. How about a walking meeting, where appropriate? It tones muscles, improves fitness, helps with circulation, aids breathing, helps reduce stress and tension, and helps you lose weight and keep it off.

WALKING IS NOT ENOUGH

Please keep in mind that I am not suggesting that you can obtain complete body fitness and health simply by walking. That is not true. That skeletal structure is held up by a whole array of muscles that are not just in your legs. To keep your skeletal structure, connective tissue and nerves from being overburdened, resulting in conditions such as back pain, knee issues or issues with other body parts, exercise your complete body. You don't have to be an athlete to do that.

Post your weight-loss and fitness goals

next to your bathroom mirror,

in your foot locker,

your wall locker,

your closet,

your car

and in the office.

Recite it,

sleep it,

sing it,

pray it

and work it.

Tell your girlfriend,
boyfriend,
husband,
wife
and anyone else you feel like telling.

Stir up some positive, goal-oriented energy.

YOUR ACTION PLAN

SIX KEYS TO WEIGHT LOSS

ACTION #1 – NO MORE EXCUSES – ELIMINATE ALL EXCUSES

Do what you say you're going to do. Not following through is a roadblock to permanent weight-loss and weight management.

ACTION #2 – TALK TO WIN – TALK ABOUT GOALS, NOT OBSTACLES

Program yourself with positive, take-charge and take-personal responsibility talk, NOT talk that focuses on external, "out-of-your-control" circumstances or people.

ACTION #3 – THINK TO WIN – DWELL ON THE POSITIVE (= GOALS TO ACCOMPLISH), NOT THE NEGATIVE (= OBSTACLES TO OVERCOME)

Dwell on positive thoughts even under negative circumstances. There are no quick fixes for weight-loss or weight management or life. Only your determination to make positive changes can make positive changes. Take command of your mind and your thoughts, and you will succeed.

ACTION #4 – EAT TO WIN – BALANCE QUANTITY AND QUALITY OF FOOD

Watch the quantity and the quality of the foods you eat. Choose healthy food that you enjoy. Eat regularly. Eat balanced meals and eat healthful snacks that satisfy. Eat fiber-rich, predominantly plant-based foods that are minimally manipulated by man (unprocessed). Drink lots of water. Avoid fast food and junk food. Take charge of the grocery store and the dining table. Take a multi-vitamin without any thought that you will be getting health from a pill. The vitamin pill – or any other pill, supplement or powder – is no replacement for healthful, close-to-nature food.

ACTION #5 – LIKE HOW YOU LOOK

Go look in the mirror, smile, and say words of praise and encouragement. You ARE your own best friend. Treat yourself that way, and then treat others the same.

ACTION #6 – MOVE

Physical fitness and weight management require a lifelong commitment of time and effort. Exercise must become one of those things that you do without question. Like bathing and brushing your teeth, once is not enough.

CHAPTER FOUR

FITNESS GOALS AND PROGRESS MEASUREMENT

"A prudent person foresees the danger ahead and takes precautions; the simpleton goes blindly on and suffers the consequences." Proverbs 22:3 – Bible, New Living Translation

In order to go from Point A to Point B, you've got to know where Point A is. You will establish your Point A in your fitness journey by measuring and testing. You will measure your:

- Body Mass Index (BMI)
- Size of your body parts
- Cardio, strength and muscle endurance
- Height and weight

BODY MASS INDEX (BMI)

Body Mass Index (BMI) is a number calculated from a person's height and weight. BMI provides a reliable indicator of body fatness for most people and is used to screen for weight categories that may lead to health problems. If, however, you are a body-builder or naturally have a big, muscular build, BMI may not work as a reliable indicator of progress. Those with a relatively large, muscular build need to understand that they have the special challenge to maintain their cardio conditioning. Otherwise, they are at a heightened risk for health issues specific to that body type.

INTERPRETATION OF BMI FOR ADULTS

For adults 20 years old and older, BMI is interpreted using standard weight status categories that are the same for all ages and for both men and women. For children and teens, on the other hand, the interpretation of BMI is both age- and sex-specific.

Standard BMI weight status categories for adults

☐ Below 18.5 is underweight.
☐ 18.5 to 24.9 is a healthy weight.
☐ 25.0 to 29.9 is overweight.
☐ 30.0 and above is obese.

EXAMPLE OF SOMEONE WHO IS 5'9" TALL

☐ 124 lbs or less is a BMI below 18.5 and is underweight.
☐ 125 lbs to 168 lbs is within a BMI range of 18.5 to 24.9 and is a healthy weight.
☐ 169 lbs to 202 lbs is within a BMI range of 25.0 to 29.9 and is overweight.
☐ 203 lbs or more is a BMI range of 30.0 or higher and is obese.

Source: Centers for Disease Control and Prevention, CDC, website: www.cdc.gov

LET'S TALK ABOUT BODY FAT

I recommend using BMI to easily get an idea of where you stand with healthy or unhealthy body fat. The body fat percentage categories below are guidelines. If you would like a quick and easy way to calculate your body fat, go to the website www.csgnetwork.com/bodyfatcalc.html. This is designed to give the approximate percentage of body fat, based on weight and waist size as compared to tables published by the American Medical Association. Just enter your present weight and waist size.

The American Council on Exercise has categorized ranges of body fat percentages as follows:

Essential fat
- Women 12-15%
- Men 2-5%

Athletes
- Women 16–20%
- Men 6–13%

Fitness
- Women 21–24%
- Men 14–17%

Acceptable
- Women 25–31%
- Men 18–25%

Obese
- Women 32%+
- Men 25%+

Essential fat values are lower than the recommended minimum body fat percentage levels. A small amount of *storage* fat is required to be available as fuel for the body in time of need. It can be dangerous to have _essential_ body fat levels as low as depicted on the chart above.

BODY MEASUREMENTS USING A TAILOR'S MEASURING TAPE

A quick and simple way to measure loss of body fat is to take body measurements with a measuring tape every four weeks as a part of your M.O.V.E.™ program. You will need a buddy to take the measurements for you. Always take body measurements on the right side of your body. We will limit the measurements to the following body parts so that you have some fast and easy indicators of your progress. Also, since you will probably be clothed for these measurements, make sure that you are wearing the same clothing for each of the measurements to ensure an accurate measurement of progress. The measurements should be taken at the same time of day, and not just after a meal or a vigorous exercise session.

NECK CIRCUMFERENCE

Your arms are relaxed at your sides in the standing position, and your neck is relaxed. Measure the smallest circumference of your neck, and note the number of inches.

ARM

Measure the arm circumference with the subject standing upright, shoulders relaxed, and the right arm extended out to the side and parallel to the ground. It is important to be certain that the muscle of the arm is not flexed or tightened, which could yield a larger and inaccurate reading. Your buddy will stand facing your right side. Place the tape around the largest part of the bicep/tricep and measure.

CHEST CIRCUMFERENCE

Your arms are relaxed and at your sides. Your buddy takes the measuring tape under your arms and around your chest where the nipples are. Relax your breathing during this measurement.

ABDOMINAL CIRCUMFERENCE

Measure abdominal circumference against the skin at the belly button. Arms are relaxed at the sides. Take a relaxed exhale and have your buddy take the measurement.

WAIST CIRCUMFERENCE

To measure your waist circumference, place a tape measure around your abdominal region just above your hip bone. Be sure that the tape is firm but not too tight. Slowly exhale and take the measurement.

ILIAC CIRCUMFERENCE

Stand and find where your upper pelvic bones protrude the most; you can feel for them on either side of your waist. Measure the circumference at this point. It could be about two inches below the navel (belly button), but can vary from person to person.

HIP CIRCUMFERENCE

Stand and find the area of your body below your navel where you are the widest. This area can vary greatly from person to person. Wrap the tape measure around your body and take the measurement.

CALF CIRCUMFERENCE

You're in the standing position. Relax your right leg and put your weight on your left leg. Now measure the calf circumference of the right at the widest point.

FITNESS TEST

It's time to test your muscle endurance, cardio and strength. All it takes are three very basic activities, push-ups, crunches or sit-ups and a one-mile run/walk. Use the results as a benchmark. You need the benchmark in order to establish reasonable, attainable goals to shoot for every four weeks of testing. For your kick-start program, test yourself every four weeks for four months. After that, you can test yourself every three months or twice a year. If you notice you're falling back to your old ways of insufficient exercise, the fitness test will let you know and become a wake-up call to get back on track.

CONDUCT THE FITNESS TEST EVENTS IN THIS ORDER:

1. Push-ups
2. Crunches or sit-ups
3. One mile run/walk

PUSH-UPS (KNEE OR REGULAR)

The push-up will test the endurance of your chest, shoulders and triceps. Rest is permitted in the up position of the push-up or by raising your rearward anatomy while in the upward push-up position. Only correct push-ups count. You have two minutes to perform as many as you can. You count the completed repetition in the up position.

CRUNCHES OR SIT-UPS

Choose regular crunches or sit-ups for this event. The sit-up measures the endurance of your abdominals and hip-flexor muscles. Perform as many as you can within two minutes. You will notice that time is really of the essence when performing this event. Keep the pace up as fast as you reasonably can. Only correct repetitions count. Resting is permitted only in the "up" position for the sit-up. There is no resting position for crunches; continue performing them until the two minutes are up, or stop prior to the two minutes if too fatigued to continue.

ONE MILE RUN/WALK

The one-mile run/walk is designed to measure your aerobic fitness and leg endurance. If, however, you do not have a measured one-mile distance, pick an approximate distance with clear beginning and ending landmarks, and always use this course for your measurement of progress. Your objective is to complete this event as fast as you reasonably can.

RECORD YOUR SCORES AND ESTABLISH YOUR FOUR-WEEK GOALS

You may need some help with establishing your goals. If you are out of shape and just starting out, you will find that, with consistency, you will make significant progress with all three events.

HOW TO ESTABLISH FITNESS GOALS

Let's say you completed the one-mile run/walk in 11 minutes. I would expect that with your next test, you will complete the mile run within a range of 9 to 10 minutes, shaving off one to two minutes of your time. You will conduct a test every four weeks for at least four months. As your fitness improves the goals will probably not be as great a difference, such as shaving off one to two minutes of your time from the mile run.

U.S. Army Fitness Test Scores for 37 to 41 Year Olds		
	Male	Female
Push-ups		
Minimum	34	13
Maximum	73	40
Sit-ups		
Minimum	38	38
Maximum	76	76
Two-mile Run		
Minimum	18:16	22:42
Maximum	13:35	17:00

YOUR ACTION PLAN

Fitness Goals and Progress Measurement

☑ Test your cardio, strength and endurance at least twice a year.

☑ Calculate your Body Mass Index, as necessary.

☑ When kick-starting a fitness program, test yourself every four weeks, calculate your BMI and weigh yourself.

☑ Have a buddy take your body measurements every four weeks to kick-start your health and fitness program.

☑ Get going now and get it in your calendar!

TRAINING-PHASE CONDITIONING DRILLS

#1 PREPARATORY TRAINING

High Jumper
Push-Up (TS* 20-45** seconds)
Sit-Up (TS 20-45** seconds)
Side-Straddle Hop
Side Bender
Knee Bender
Stationary Run

#2 CONDITIONING TRAINING

Push-UP (varied hand positions)
   (TS 30-60 seconds)
Supine Bicycle
High Jumper
Sit-Up (all types)
   (TS 30-60 seconds)
The Engine or Cross-Country Skiier
All-Fours Run (stationary)

#3 MAINTENANCE TRAINING

Ski Jump
Sit-Ups (all types) (TS 30-60 seconds)
Push-Up (varied hand positions) (TS 30-60 seconds)
Mule Kick
Flutter Kick
The Engine
The Swimmer

*TS = timed set

** Because of a lower level of fitness, 45 seconds will usually be the upper limit.

Source: FM 21-20, Physical Fitness Training, US Department of the Army, p. 7-18, 30 September 1992

CHAPTER FIVE

Stretches

There are many views about stretching and its benefits. If done properly, stretching can be a relaxing and stress relieving experience. Some say that we should stretch before exercising. Others say we should stretch after exercising and still others emphasize stretching before and after. There is no substantial evidence about the benefits of stretching as it pertains to exercise or that it helps prevent injury. If you are involved in high-impact sports or athletic activity requiring the use of lots of agility, stretching could result in creating instability and actually result in injury.

My main concern is too much precious time is spent focusing on stretching and thereby neglecting the cardio and strength training which is a higher priority. Performing all movement exercises, be it strength training or cardio, results in promoting flexibility.

Stretch briefly between exercises. Please remember that you may want to leave stretching out altogether from time to time when performing a circuit routine that combines the cardio and strength training, because you want to maximize the cardio and muscle endurance benefit.

We will focus on a few basic stretches.

ARMS AND SHOULDERS

Take your right arm and place it across your chest parallel to the ground. With your left hand, reach over and grab your right elbow. Now gently pull your right arm across your chest with your left hand. Hold for 15 to 20 seconds. Switch arms and perform the same stretch.

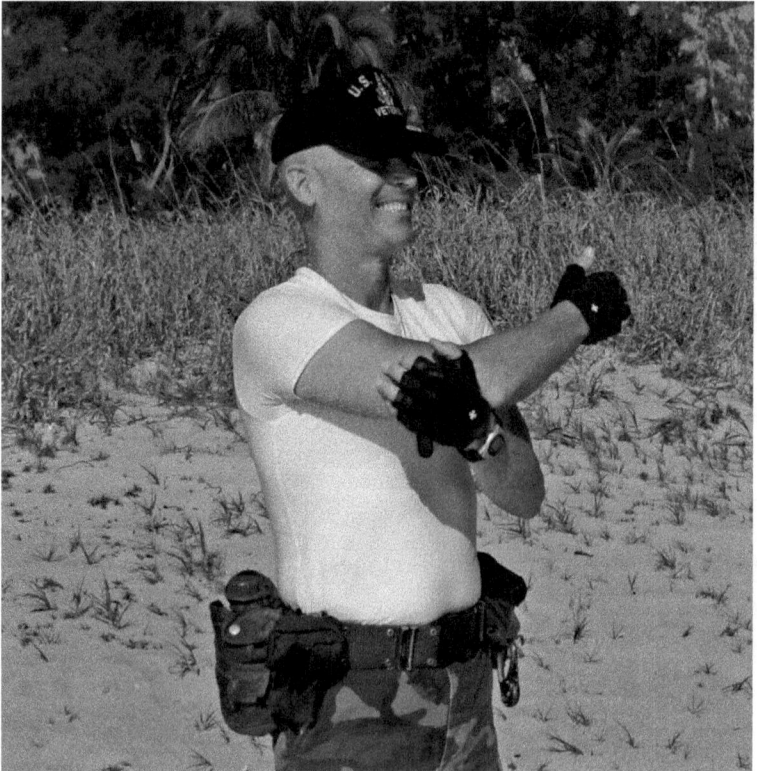

TRICEPS AND UPPER BACK

In the standing position with your feet shoulder-width apart, raise your right hand to the sky, then bend your elbow and place your right hand behind your back. Reach up over your head with your left hand and grab your right elbow. Now pull your right arm downward behind your back for a gentle stretch. Reverse arms and do it again. Hold for 15 to 20 seconds for each arm.

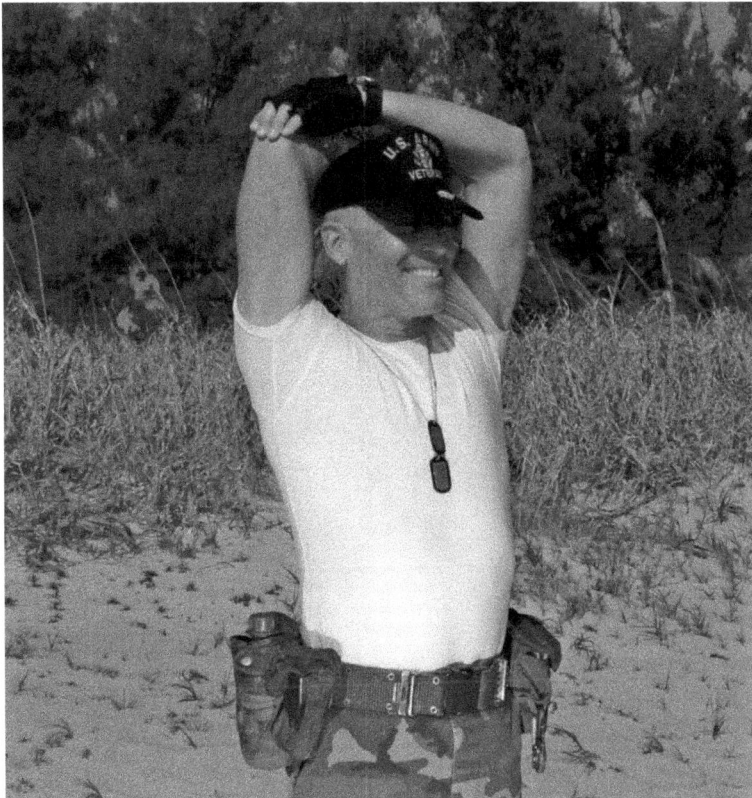

FOREARM STRETCH

After you've knocked out all those push-ups and pull-ups, you may experience some tightness in your forearms. This stretch will help to relieve the tightness. Reach your right arm out in front of you with your palm facing up as if you are making a hand signal for someone to stop. Reach over with your left hand and grab your right hand at the fingertips and gently pull back on your fingers. Hold for 15 to 20 seconds and then switch arms. For a variation, try this stretch with the fingers facing downward and then pull back with the other hand.

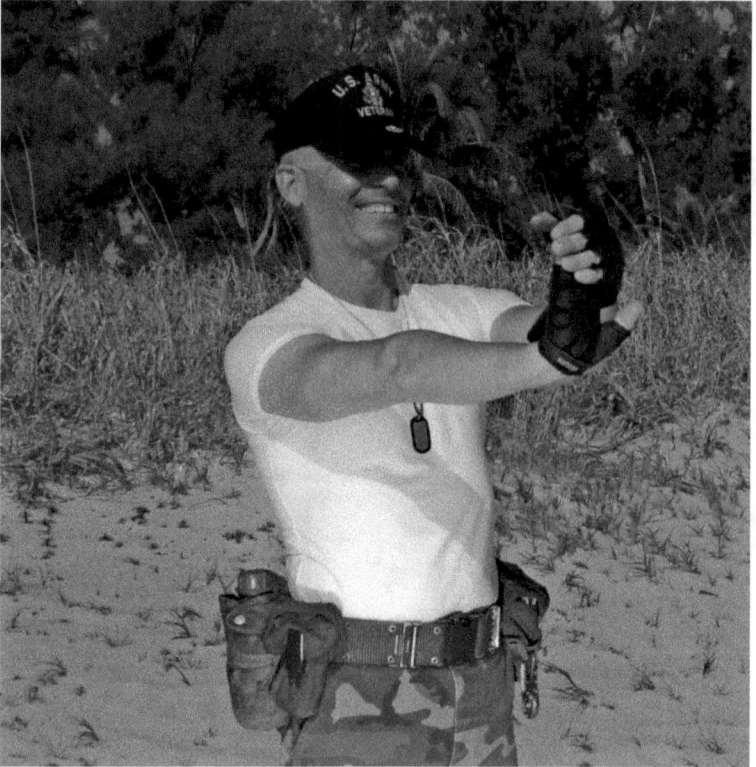

QUAD STRETCH

In the standing position, bend your right knee backward and grab your foot at the ankle with your right hand. Pull your foot to your butt while keeping your other leg straight and both legs close together. Hold for 15 to 20 seconds. Then switch sides and do the same. For support you can put the free hand against a tree, wall or on a rail.

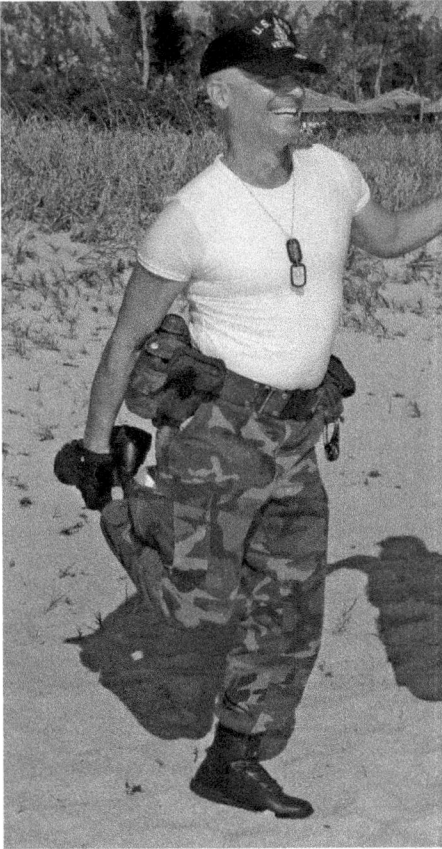

HAMSTRING STRETCH

In the standing position, extend your right leg forward and your left leg is back. Both legs are only about two feet apart, which means this is not a wide position for your legs. Now, while bending the left leg as a lever and your right leg is straight with knee locked, bend down towards your right leg and reach for the toes. You are stretching the hamstring of your right leg. To leverage that stretch, simply bend the left knee; the more you bend the left knee, the greater the stretch. No bouncing! Hold that stretch for 15 to 20 seconds. Switch positions of your legs and repeat the stretch.

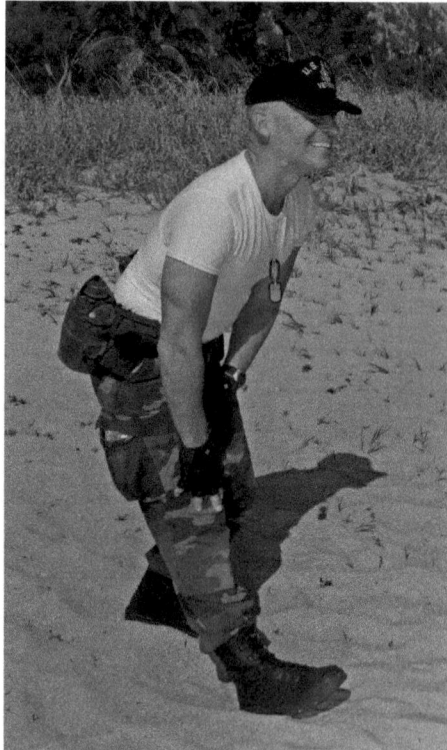

GROIN STRETCH (SEATED)

Sit on the ground with the bottoms of your feet together. Spread your legs with knees bent to have the bottoms of your feet touching. Place your hands around your feet and hold them together. Now bend forward and place your elbows on your knees and gently push downward with your elbows while keeping your head up. Hold for 15 to 20 seconds.

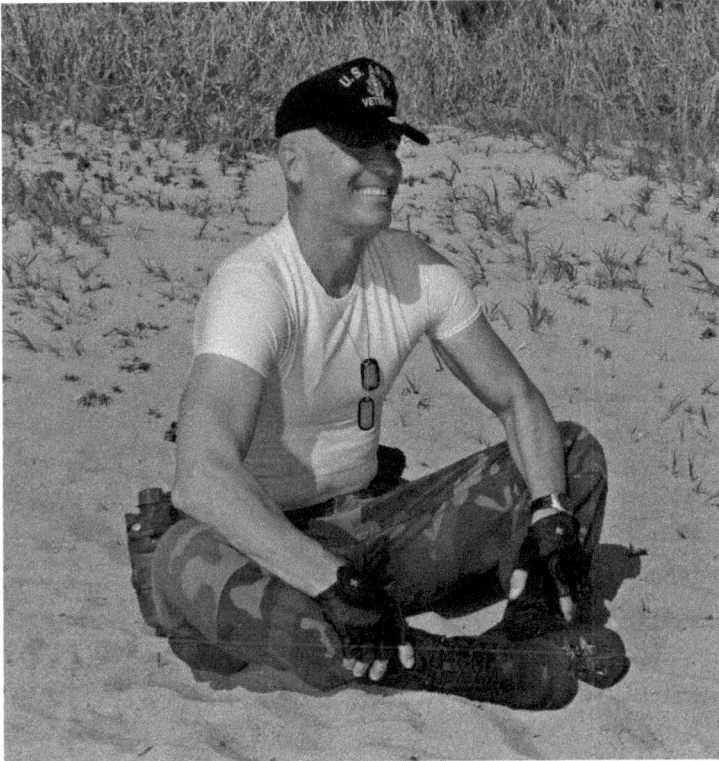

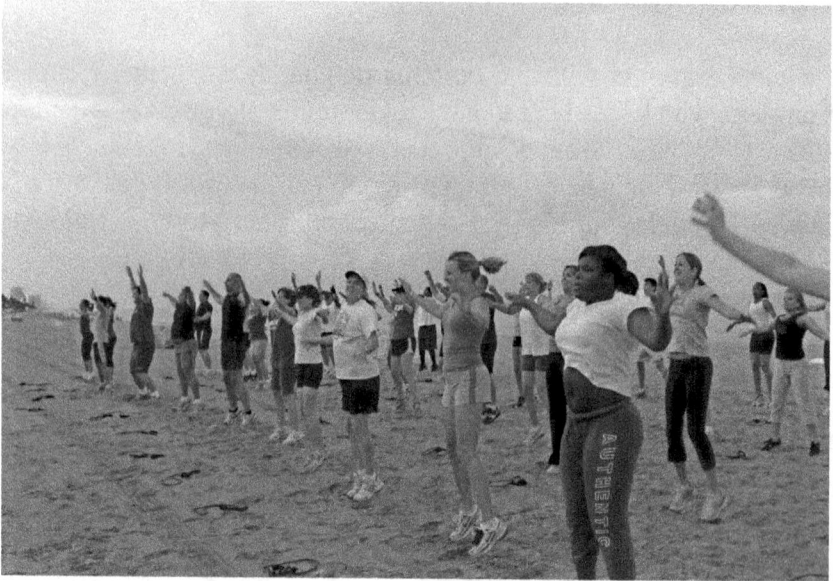

Beach Boot Camp on
Fort Lauderdale Beach, Florida.

More photos at www.beachbootcamp.net

CHAPTER SIX

NATURAL BODY WEIGHT EXERCISES

UPPER BODY

Upper body strength training without weights demonstrates the portability and flexibility of the human body when it comes to staying in shape. From a health standpoint, you do not need one single piece of equipment or some special place to stay lean and strong. Whether it's in your living room, bedroom, hotel room, on the patio, in the yard, the break room at work or in your office, you can immediately enjoy taking care of your strength training.

The following upper body natural body weight exercises are a few basics to get you started and get you in shape.

REGULAR PUSH-UP

Let's move on to the best and most complete upper body exercise in the world. It's the push-up. All right, now get down with me for this one. Let's do it! Get down on all fours. Your feet are together, your body is straight. Your arms are a little more than shoulder-width apart and are spread in line with your chest. Go down to a 90 degree break in your elbows and come back up. Now, wasn't that easy? Yeah, I know. For a lot of you out there, it's pretty strenuous. That's OK. If you find you can only go down partially, you will still be working those muscles and you will get stronger and eventually be able go all the way down. I recommend to my clients to practice the regular push-up even though they cannot go all the way down and push their body back up. This approach is better than just performing knee push-ups.

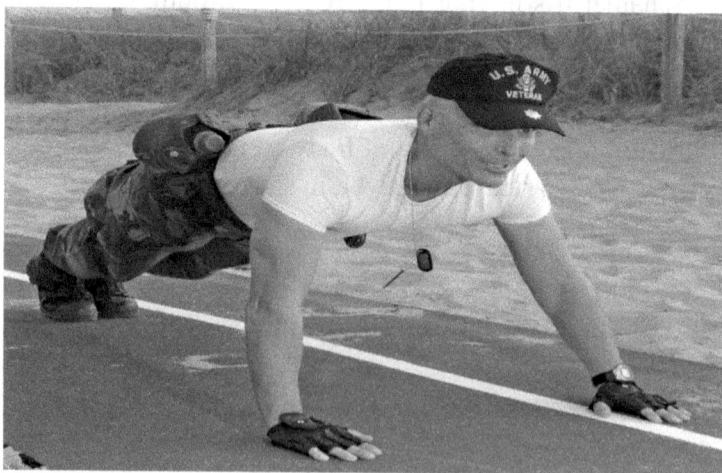

REGULAR DIPS

I know you ladies are always especially interested in working the triceps to look really good in that sleeveless dress. I've got a solution. It's called the dip. You will need a sturdy object like a chair or bench or rail that is anywhere from one to three feet off of the ground. Have a seat on the bench or chair and place your hands on each side of your body as close as you can with your fingers facing forward and curled over the edge of the bench. Your legs are about shoulder width apart with a greater than ninety degree bend. Raise your rearward anatomy off of the bench and lower your body while keeping your back close to the bench, both while going down and coming back up.

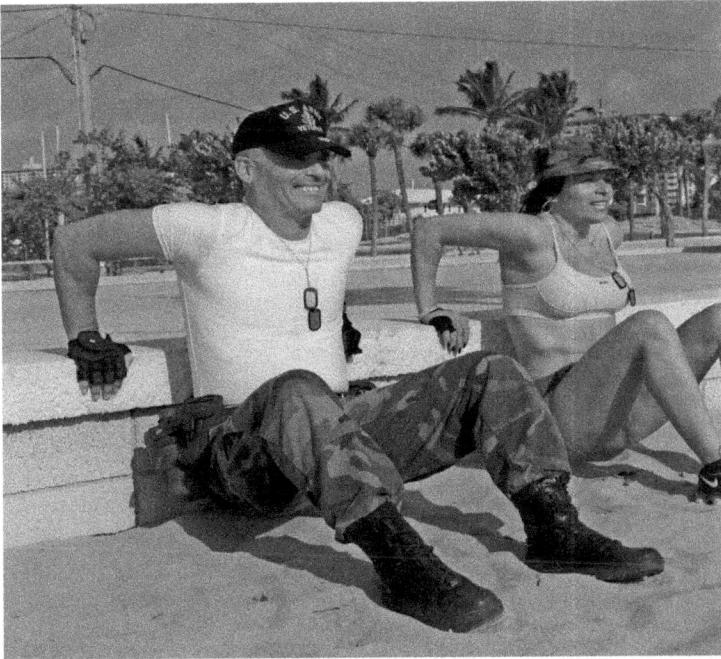

STRAIGHT LEG DIPS

Get in the same position as with the regular dips. This time, raise your right leg with knee locked and parallel to the ground. Knock out five reps just for fun. Notice the difference compared with the regular dips? Switch and raise the left leg this time. This gets me excited just writing about it! I know how good it feels!

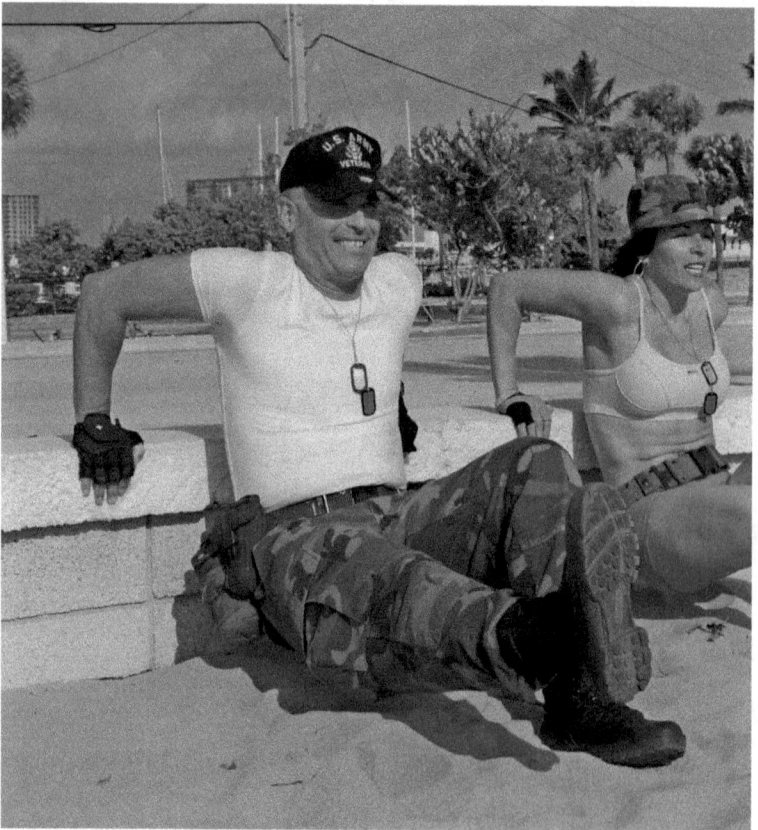

Upper Body Workout and Reps Guide			
Exercises	Beginner	Intermediate	Advanced
Regular Push-up	2 - 20	20 - 30	30 - 100
Wide Push-up	2 - 15	15 - 25	25 - 60
Tricep Push-up	2 - 8	8 - 20	20 - 50
4-count Push-up	2 - 5	8 - 20	20 - 40
Knee Push-ups, 45 Degrees	10 - 20	20 - 60	60 - 100
Knee Push-ups, 90 Degrees	10 - 20	20 - 60	60 - 100
Regular Pull-up	0 - 5	5 - 10	10 - 25
Reverse Pull-up	0 - 5	5 - 15	15 - 30
Hands-together Tricep Pull-up	0 - 3	3 - 10	10 - 20
Extra Wide Pull-up	0 - 2	2 - 5	5 - 15
Cliffhangers	0 - 2	2 - 10	10 - 20
Assisted Pull-ups	3 - 10	10 - 30	30 - 40
Straight Leg Inclines	2 - 8	8 - 20	20 - 40
Regular Dips	5 - 15	15 -40	40 - 100
Straight Leg Dips, each leg	5 - 10	10 - 20	20 - 40

For a complete demonstration of all the exercises listed in the chart above, see my book, *Change Made Easy - Your Basic Training Orders to Excellent Physical and Mental Health.*

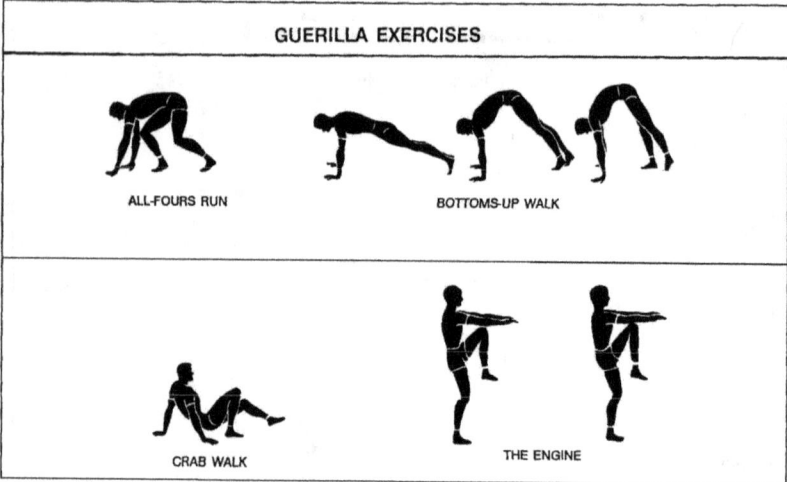

GUERILLA EXERCISES

ALL-FOURS RUN

BOTTOMS-UP WALK

CRAB WALK

THE ENGINE

Source: FM 21-20, Physical Fitness Training, US Department of the Army, p. 7-23, 30 September 1992

CHAPTER SEVEN

RESISTANCE BAND STRENGTH TRAINING

UPPER BODY

I want to introduce you to the most portable and affordable piece of equipment you can use for your workouts anywhere, anytime. It's called the resistance band or tube. It is an oversized rubber band with handles on each end for your hands. There are many manufacturers out there. I prefer the bands by the company, SPRI. There are six levels of resistance, all color coded:

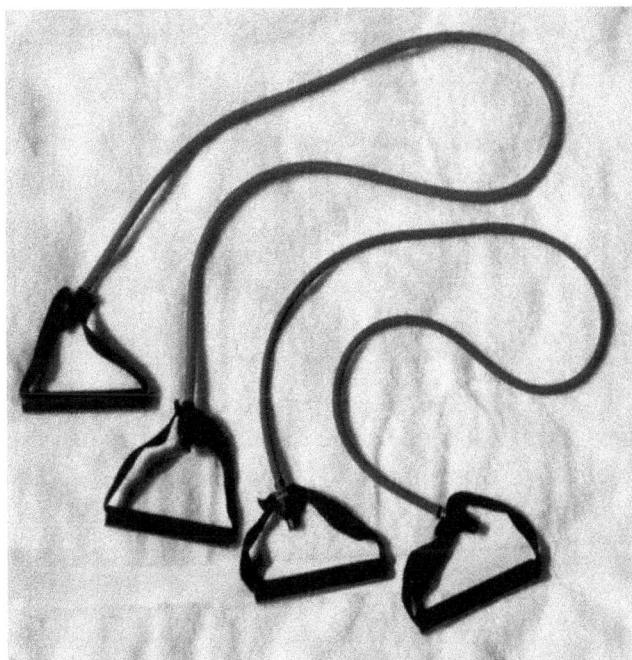

WHICH RESISTANCE BAND/TUBE IS RIGHT FOR YOU?

You need to go by your *current* strength and fitness level, not by what you would *like* to be in order to work your muscles effectively and to prevent injuries.

- **Lavender - very light** - rehab, medical conditions and frail people.

- **Yellow - light** - children, rehab, some women and seniors, 2-5 lbs.

- **Green - medium** - average (inactive) women and some older men, 5-10 lbs.

- **Red - heavy** - average men and active, fairly strong women, 11-16 lbs.

- **Blue - extra-heavy** - active men and very strong women, 17-22 lbs.

- **Purple/black - ultra-heavy** - strong men or women body-builders, 23-30 lbs.

Choosing a band will depend upon the type of workout you are doing. If you are performing high reps of 50 to 100 you will probably use at least one level down compared to performing just 10 to 20 reps per set. Your fatigue level while performing circuit training (combined cardio and strength training) will also play a roll when choosing a resistance band. You may or may not choose a high resistance level depending upon how intense you conduct your circuit training.

BICEP CURLS

Grab each handle with your left and right hand. Your feet are shoulder width apart and you are standing firmly on the band with the band in the center of your shoes. Bend your knees slightly to stabilize your lower back with your palms facing out and your arms extended down. Pull the band up to your shoulder joint and resist it going down.

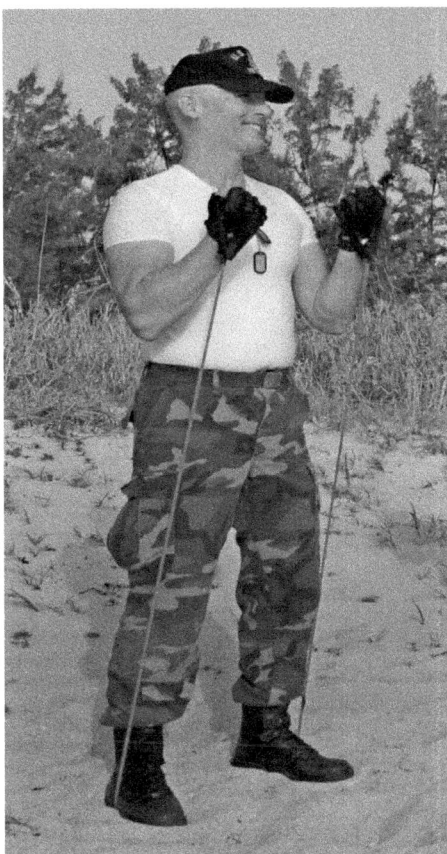

UPRIGHT ROW

Grab each handle with your left and right hand. Two feet on the band, your feet are shoulder width apart with a slight bend in the knees to stabilize your lower back. With both wrists hanging down, pull the band up to your shoulder joint while maintaining your wrists in the down position and then back to the starting position while resisting it going down. Let's practice. And one, two, three, four, five.

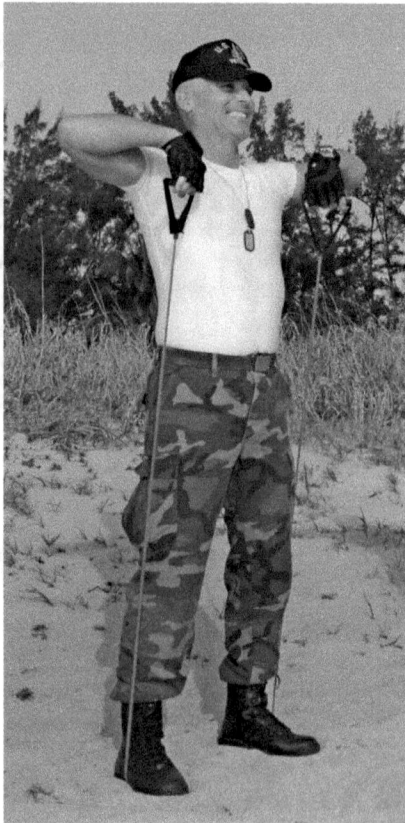

SHOULDER PRESS

Grab each handle with your left and right hand. Your left foot is on the band in the center of the shoe. Step through the band/tube with your right foot. Bring your arms up to a ninety degree break in your elbows. Your wrists are straight and the band is behind the arms.

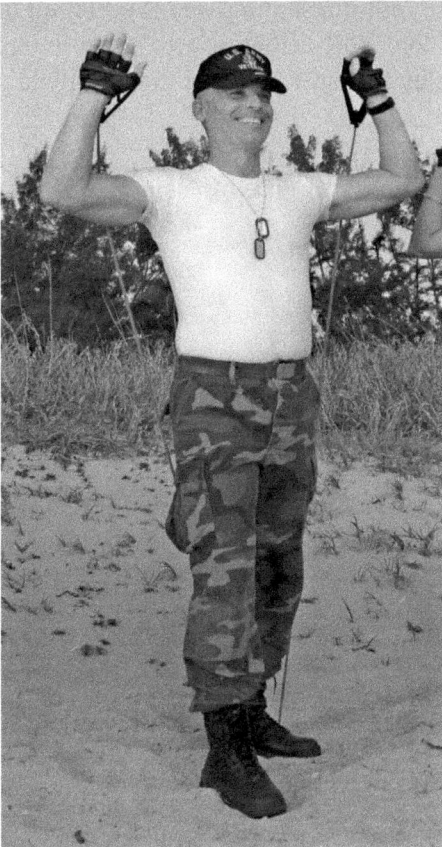

STANDING ROW

Grab each handle with your left and right hand. This next exercise will really demonstrate the versatility of the resistance band and how to incorporate your environment into the workout. Wrap the band around a tree or pole. We're going to perform a standing row exercise. Your band is wrapped around the tree. Get some resistance in the band with palms facing inward and an exaggerated bend in your knees to stabilize your lower back. Your back is straight and arms completely extended for the starting position. Pull back on the band in line with your chest and resist it going all the way back out. Find a distance that will allow you to have enough resistance to work your muscles and still perform the complete range of motion. That's one rep.

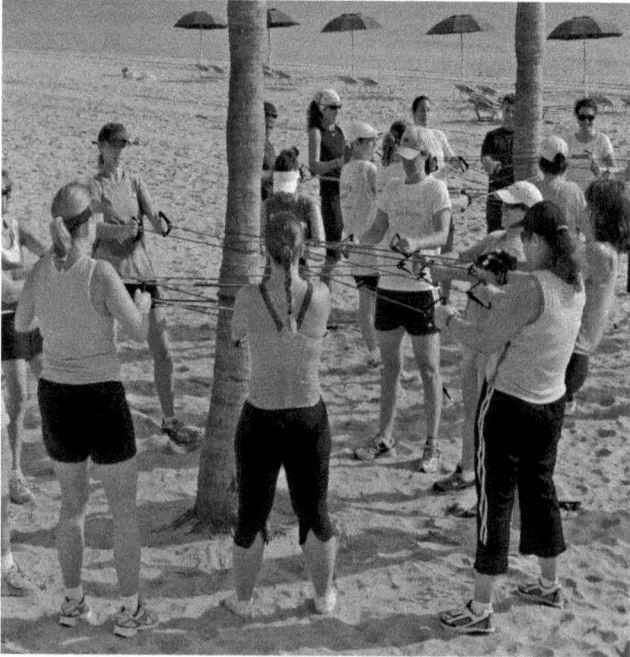

STANDING TRICEPS PUSH

Grab each handle with your left and right hand. Let's move on to another great triceps exercise with the resistance band. It's called the standing triceps push. Take the band in your right hand and place the other end on the ground in front of your right foot. Place your right foot six to eight inches into the band and firmly onto to the band with the ball of your foot so that it doesn't slip. Now step forward with your left foot, while keeping your right foot on the band. Take your right hand with the band and bring it up behind your head. The starting position is with the hand lowered behind your head. Push up on the band until the arm is completely extended. That's one rep.. Switch hands and feet and do the same thing with the left side of your body.

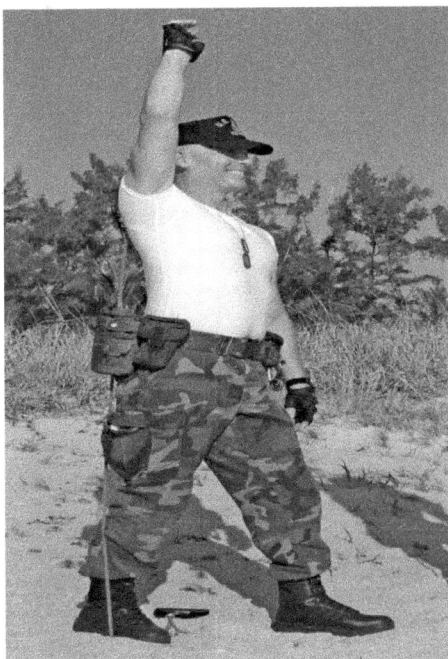

STANDING ROW WITH THE THERA-BAND LATEX RE-SISTIVE EXERCISE BAND

As with the standing row using the resistance tube wrapped around the tree the theraband offers the same kind of flexibility and portability. This type of band has no handles so you wrap each end around your hands and hold tightly.

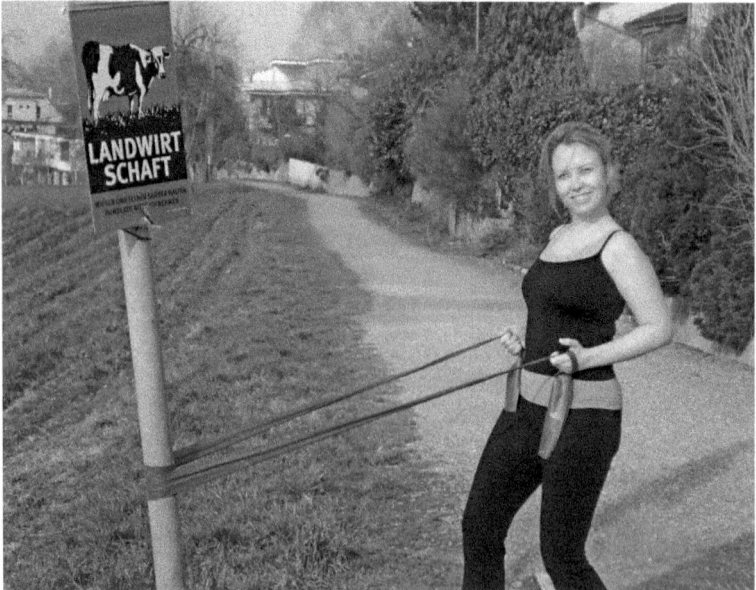

PRONE POSITION EXERCISES WITH THE THERA-BAND

The sky is truly the limit with these exercises. Have you ever seen such a smile?

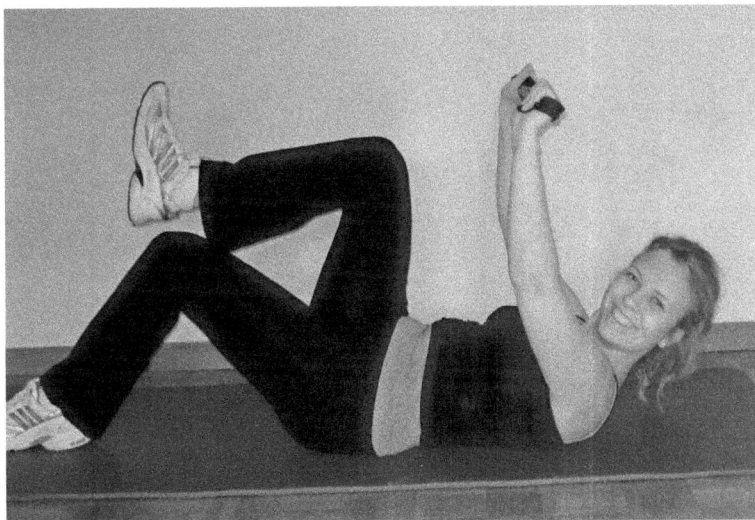

Resistance Band Upper Body Workout Reps Guide

Exercises	Beginner	Intermediate	Advanced
Bicep Curls	5 - 30	30 - 60	60 - 100
Upright Row	5 - 40	40 - 60	60 - 100
Shoulder Press	3 - 10	10 - 15	15 - 40
Front Raise	5 - 10	10 - 15	15 - 20
Side Lateral Raise	5 - 10	10 - 15	15 - 20
Standing Row	10 - 40	40 - 70	70 - 100
Standing Triceps Push	5 - 10	10 - 20	20 - 30
Reverse Curls	4 - 15	15 - 20	20 - 40
Partner Assisted Standing Arm Curl	10 - 20	20 - 30	30 - 60

CHAPTER EIGHT

WITHOUT WEIGHTS

LOWER BODY EXERCISES

BODY PARTS WORKED:
HIPS, THIGHS, BUTT, QUADS AND HAMSTRINGS

The strength training exercises described in this chapter will equip you to work your lower body completely independent of exercise equipment. For the busy person, these exercises are optimal. Many of these can even be performed within the constrains of a work cubicle. Imagine calling a brief time out in your cubicle "jungle" with all heads popping up and then performing a squat or some other exercise together. This may very well be as entertaining as Meerkat Manor on Animal Planet. Add some music and MTV will be calling. What a way to combine team building, having fun and it will certainly loosen up the atmosphere and reduce stress. By getting that blood flowing from all that sedentary work, it'll even promote increased performance.

SQUATS

Your feet are shoulder width apart with your arms on your hips or hands together with elbows bent and your head up and upper body in a natural upright position – not the bending over forward ski position. Bend your knees to a 90 degree break making sure that your knee does not go past your big toe. Then bring your body back up to the upright position. That's one repetition.

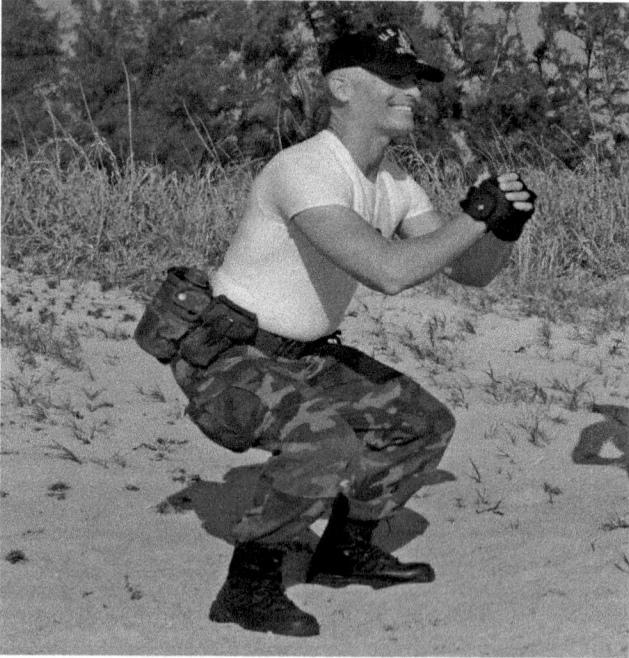

WALKING LUNGES

Pretend you are carrying two full buckets of water to emphasize good posture of your upper body in the upright position. What I want you to do is step forward with your right foot to the point where your knees are bent at 90 degrees. Your knee of the forward leg should not go past your big toe. Pause briefly and then step all the way through with your left leg. Pause briefly. Now continue this exercise. As a matter of fact, why not just go for a walk like this? Who knows? You may strike up some interesting conversation along the way.

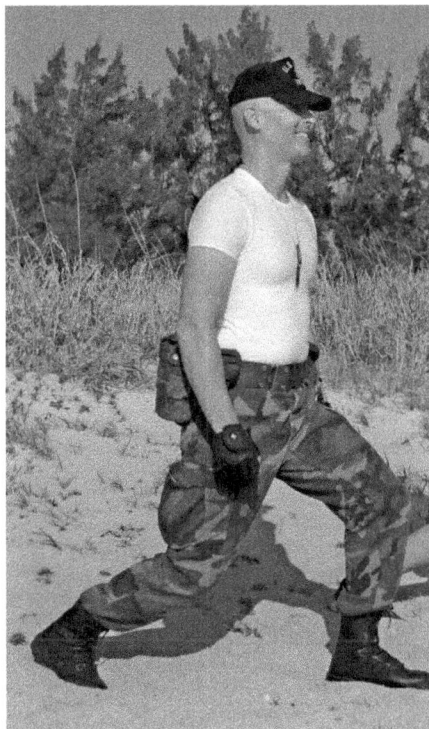

DIRTY DOGS

Get down on all fours with your head facing forward. You will need your visualization skills for this. Imagine it's time to take Fido around the block for those customary stops along the way. You now move up to the first tree and Fido stops and raises his leg smartly to take care of business. This is a great opportunity to mark your territory. When taking on any project or task in life, it's essential that you take ownership (= mark your territory). Now raise your right leg with the knee bent just like Fido and lower it again. That's one rep. For example, do twenty reps with the right leg and switch off and do twenty with the left. Now here's a test question for you. Why do you want to perform the same number of reps for both legs? Hint: How would a lopsided butt look? Spare me the thought!

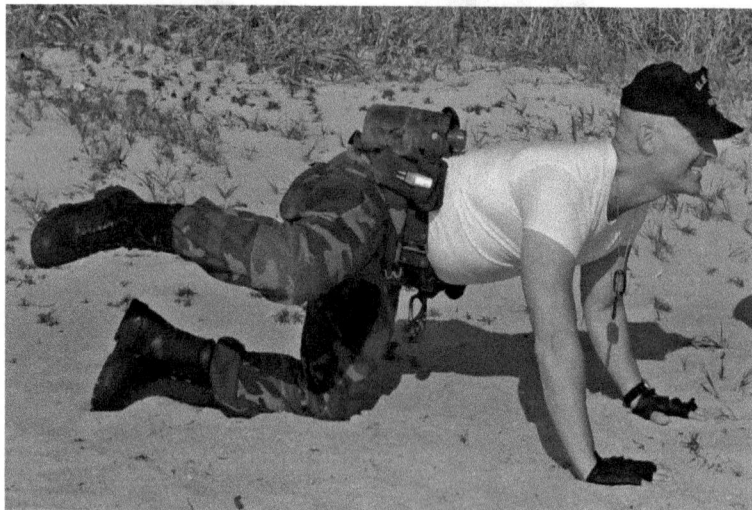

LEG THRUSTS

Get down on all fours facing forward. Take your right leg and thrust it straight back while holding it parallel to the ground with the toes pointed downward, then thrust the leg back to the position where you attempt to touch your chest with your knee. That is one rep. Count the rep with the straight leg position. Switch legs to work the other side. For example, do twenty reps with the right leg, then do twenty with the left. As with many of those body weight exercises there are many variations that can be performed. This is just one of them.

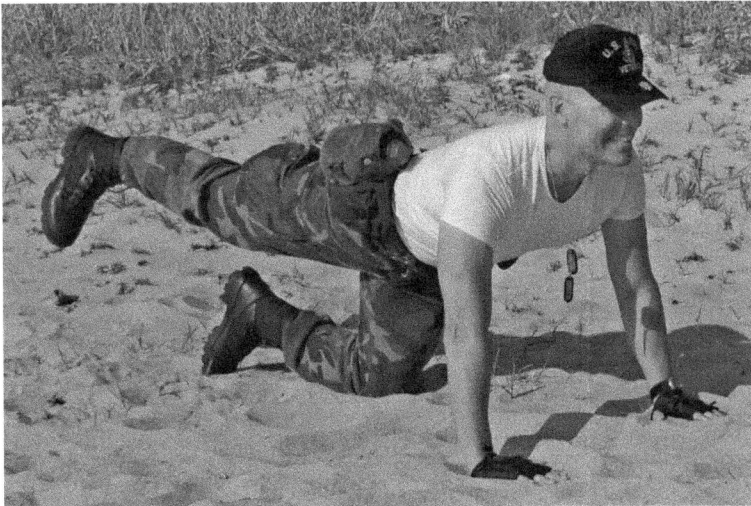

ALTERNATING SIDE LEG RAISES (4-COUNT EXERCISE)

Stand with feet shoulder width apart and with bent elbows and hands together just about chest high. Now squat down to the point where your legs are at a 90 degree angle. Make sure your knee does not go past your big toe. Here's the 4-count: ONE, squat to 90 degrees; TWO, lift (not kick) your left leg out to about hip height to the extended position with knees locked; THREE, back to the squat position; FOUR, lift (not kick) your right leg to about hip height while keeping it straight. That is one rep. 10 reps are a good number per set.

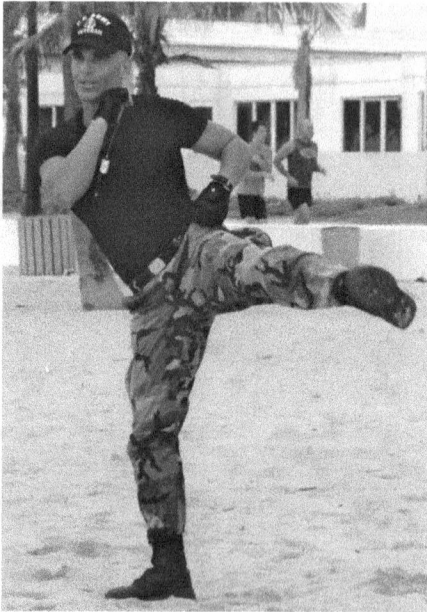

Lower Body Workout Reps Guide

Exercises	Beginner	Intermediate	Advanced
Squats	20 - 40	40 - 100	100 - 200
Standing Lunges, each leg	5 - 20	20 - 60	60 - 100
Dirty Dogs, each leg	5 - 10	10 - 40	40 - 80
Leg Thrusts, each leg	5 - 20	20 - 50	50 - 80
Standing Crunches, each leg	10 - 30	30 - 60	60 - 100
Alternating Side Leg Raise (Lift)	10 - 15	15 - 30	30 - 70

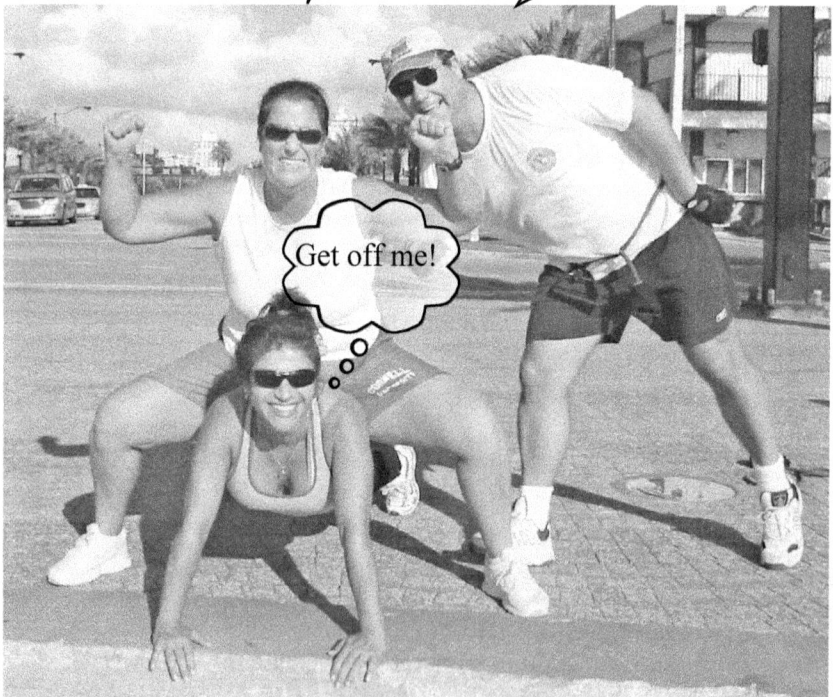

Who said exercise is all work and no play?

CHAPTER NINE

Jump, Kick and Punch

BODY PARTS WORKED:
HEART, LUNGS, BUTT, HIPS, THIGHS, CALVES, QUADS, HAMSTRINGS, ARMS

The number and variations of body weight exercises are limitless. The following exercises are not included in the upper and lower body weight exercises because I consider them to be in a category of their own. This does not mean that you won't be working the upper or lower body. The opposite is true. Remember, our bodies are designed to work in sync. These basic supplemental exercises add to your arsenal of body weight exercises which is what you need to keep your program interesting, fun and health focused.

JUMPING JACKS

A callisthenic workout is never complete without jumping jacks. Stand with feet together and arms at your sides. You're going to need a little bounce for this one. Jump to the spread leg position and land your feet back on the ground while you bring your arms together over your head (arms are raised and extended over your head). Then immediately jump back to the starting position with feet together while bringing your arms back down to your sides. This is a smooth motion. Jump out. Then jump back to the starting position. That is one repetition. Perform 50 to 100 reps. Of course you can start out with less, if you feel the need. This is a high impact exercise . If you have any medical issues with your knees or ankles, please consult your physician. Try modifying the exercise by spreading your legs partially and not jumping as high if you have a medical issue that allows you to modify the exercise.

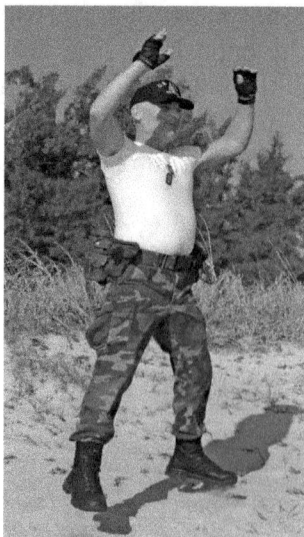

WIND MILLS

Stand with your feet wider than shoulder width apart and arms extended parallel to the ground, out to your sides and palms facing down with elbows locked. Bend over and take your right hand diagonally across your body and reach for your left foot while extending your left arm pointing towards the sky and then back to the starting position with both arms extend out and parallel to the ground. In the starting position you're not bent over but standing erect between each repetition. Perform 10 to 20 reps.

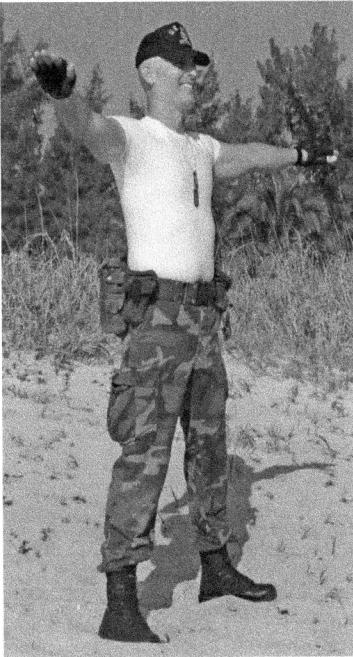

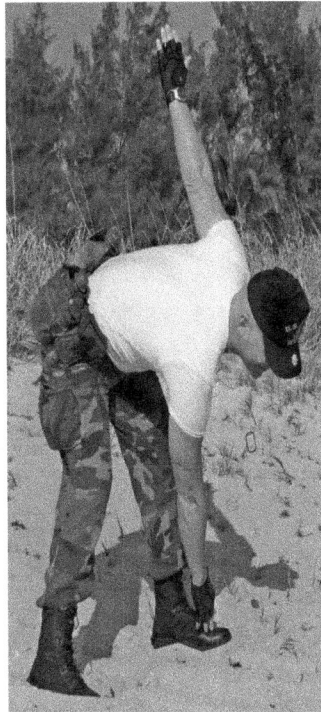

KICK

Your right leg is back. Your left leg is forward. Perform a snap kick with the right leg by thrusting it out and kicking about kneecap high and then back to the starting position. That is one repetition. Switch legs to work the other side. For example, if you are performing thirty reps, work first one leg with all thirty and then the other. Count the reps with the leg in the extended (kick) position. Perform 30 to 60 reps with each leg.

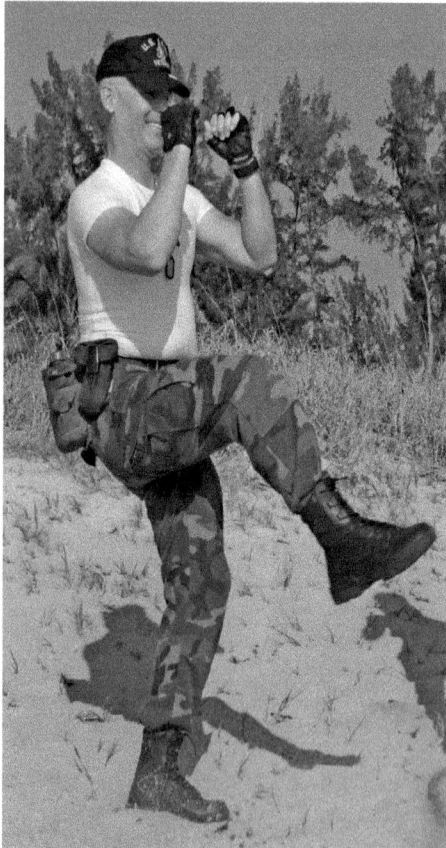

SIDE PUNCH

Your legs are shoulder width apart and fists are clenched and positioned in front of your face. Now punch your right fist to the left and snap it back to the starting position. Then punch your left fist to the right and snap it back to the starting position. Note that you are swiveling your hips for each punch and looking in the direction of your punch. This is a four count exercise. ONE; your right arm punches out to the left; TWO, your right arm is back to the starting position; THREE, your left arm punches out to the right; FOUR, your left arm is back to the starting position. That is one repetition. Perform 40 to 80 reps per set.

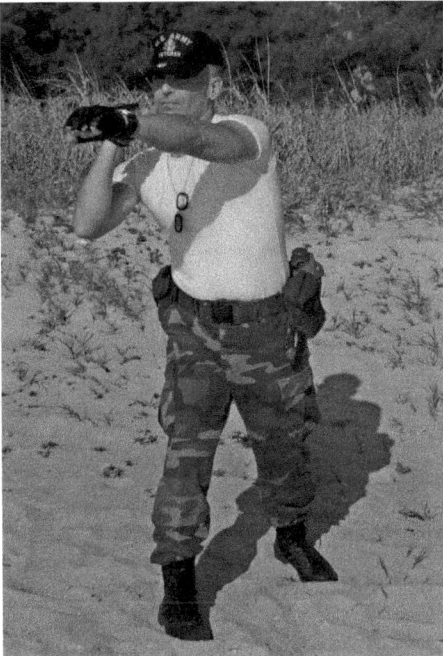

TOE RAISERS

Your feet are shoulder width apart with arms raised as if you are under arrest. Now reach down and touch your stomach, then your toes, then your stomach and back up to the starting position. This is a four count exercise. ONE, touch your stomach; TWO, touch your toes; THREE, touch your stomach; FOUR, back to the starting position with both arms raised above your head and extended. That is one repetition. Perform 50 to 100 reps. Some of you are asking, "Why toe raisers?" Well, you can add a calf raise to this exercise by taking it up on your toes when you reach for the sky. Now you know why they're called toe raisers.

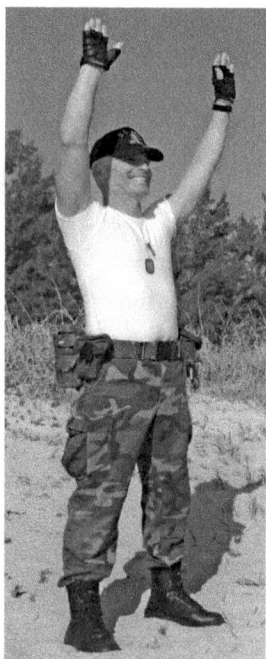

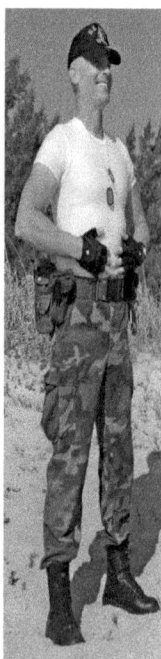

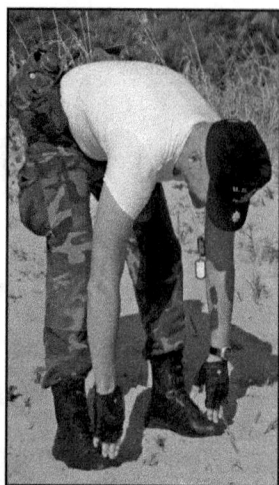

CHAPTER TEN

CARDIO AND AGILITY DRILLS

BODY PARTS WORKED:
LUNGS, HEART, HIPS, THIGHS, CALVES, BUTT, ABS AND LOWER BACK

It's time to add some fun and games to your workout with some cardio and agility drills. Always consider your physical activity a dynamic and not static process. Make it a game. Think variety. Incorporate your environment into your workout. Though these drills call for the use of cones, you could use stones are even trees and bushes or chairs to run around. Always keep safety in mind.

BACKPEDAL/SPRINT DRILL (STAGGERED CONES)

Six cones will be needed for this drill. Place one cone as the starting point and the other five are placed like spokes in a wheel at different lengths (10 to 20 yards) from the starting cone and each of them about five yards apart. Each of the five cones will be placed at the 10, 12, 1 and 2 o'clock positions. Sprint to the 10 o'clock cone and backpedal back to the starting cone. Do this with each cone in the "spoke" until all are completed.

ZIGZAG SPRINT DRILL WITH CONES

Using six cones, stagger them in such a way that you will have to zigzag around each of them in order. This is a sprinting drill. Each cone should be about 5 yards apart. You will sprint around each cone until you have zigzagged through all the cones and then back again. The cones will be placed in two rows.

BOX DRILL WITH CONES

Using four cones form a box on your lawn. The cones can be about 25 yards apart although you my vary that distance as you like. You are standing at the first cone. You will sprint to the second cone. You will perform a lateral or sideways move to the third cone. You will back pedal to the fourth cone. You will sprint back to the first cone. Please note that you can simply just sprint to each cone or you can mix and match your own moves between each of the cones.

SUICIDES

This is a simple drill with a high cardio impact. Place one cone as the starting point and the other cone anywhere from 20 to 50 yards out. Sprint out and back, out and back, out and back, and so forth. I think you get the point. You can simply make this one a timed event with everyone at their own pace. When performing this as a group the great benefit is that no one really ever falls behind.

As a matter of fact, you really can't tell who's ahead and who's behind. Regardless of fitness level all team members will enjoy a great cardio blast with this drill. I'm sure you'll notice the fatigue very quickly on this one.

FORWARD-BACK-LEFT-RIGHT

This can be done in a group with a group leader guide or by yourself. The guide leader will call the signals randomly to change direction. Don't run into any trees or fall in a ditch going backwards! The commands are simple: FORWARD, BACK, LEFT, RIGHT. The commands FORWARD and BACK simply mean to run forward and backward. The commands LEFT and RIGHT mean run sideways to the left and to the right. This is lots of fun and a great way to work on the agility and the lower body. How long? As long as the guide leader is yelling out commands. The leader can either face the group and give hand signals as well or he or she can join in with the group and shout out the commands.

RUN FORREST RUN!

I'm sure most of you have seen the movie "Forrest Gump." Once Forrest started running, he didn't know when to stop. For most of us out there, it's more like not knowing when to start. I had to specifically mention running. What I mean is anything that leaves the realm of simply walking. Keep in mind that running (jogging) is a great way to work the heart, lungs, butt, hips, thighs, quads, hamstrings and much more.

LEARN TO THROTTLE YOUR RUNNING PACE

Before ever stopping, try throttling it down to a slower running or jogging pace first. This works on two things: your mental strength and it keeps you on the run. Unless you are sprinting, your upper body should be relaxed and only your legs and lungs should be working. No feet dragging or pavement pounding is permitted unless you have a sudden urge to hear me say, "Drop and give me twenty!" Foot dragging or scraping or foot pounding is a recipe for injuries to connective tissue in your lower body. Your stride and your body mechanics should be smooth. You land on your heels and roll across your foot. You're not really going to be thinking about this when you run. Just check yourself every now and then for smooth, efficient running mechanics.

Your breathing – as with all exercises - should be natural and should not be heard, and the mouth should not be making some unnatural forms that you've seen in some of those workout videos or in the gym. You're getting some of the Health Colonel's philosophy about breathing.

YOUR BODY IS DESIGNED TO RUN

Oh, and by the way, your body was designed to run, contrary to some of the things you may have heard. The latest research has determined the gluts – that's that

rearward anatomy, also known as the butt – are not really working when walking. I want to emphasize the running because it is also working the complete lower body to include the lower back and abs. (Source: NewScientist.com: July 30, 2007 "Duplicate genes help humans go the extra mile," by Roxanne Khamsi; Discovermagazine.com, May 28, 2006, "Born To Run, Biomechanical research reveals a surprising key to the survival of our species: Humans are built to outrun nearly every other animal on the planet over long distances." by Ingfei Chen)

RUNNING TIMES FOR BEGINNER, INTERMEDIATE AND ADVANCED

Run Forrest run!			
	Beginner	**Intermediate**	**Advanced**
Run 1 Mile	11:00 - 18:00	8:00 - 11:00	5:00 - 8:00
Run 2 Miles	16:00 - 30:00	14:00 - 16:00	10:00 - 14:00

BACKPEDAL

Who says you always have to run or walk forward? There are actually backward track races. Now, I do have to admit that the falls during these races are quite spectacular and a sight to see. Ouch! Backpedaling is a great way to recruit those lower body muscles in a different way. Just make sure that you use your peripheral vision so that you don't run into that tree or signpost and definitely do not run backwards (or forwards) in traffic. I provided some great entertainment during a group class on the beach when I ran right into a palm tree. Don't worry. No injuries except for my pride.

TUG-O-WAR

Remember those days in school or summer camp when you would engage in a tug-o-war competition with a rope? Well, this happens to be an exercise (or game) that you can't do alone. You'll need a rope of special tug-o-war material with loops. Do an internet search and you will find lots of options.

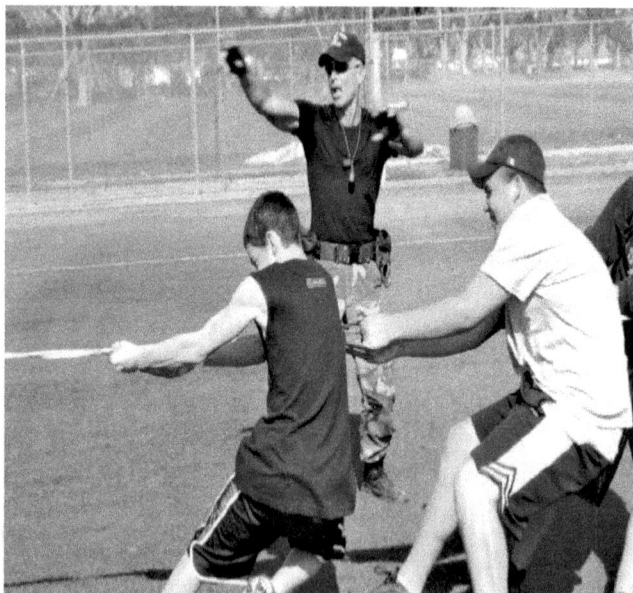

Run, Jump, Kick, Punch Workout Guides			
Exercises	**Beginner**	**Intermediate**	**Advanced**
Jumping Jacks	10 - 30	30 - 50	50 - 100
Wind Mills, 4 count	5 - 15	15 - 30	30 - 80
Snap Kick, each leg	10 - 30	30 - 60	60 - 100
Side Punch Drill, 4 count	10 - 30	30 - 60	60 - 100
Toe Raisers, 4 count	20 - 40	40 - 70	70 - 100
Run 1 Mile	11:00 - 18:00	8:00 - 11:00	5:00 - 8:00
Run 2 Miles	16:00 - 30:00	14:00 - 16:00	10:00 - 14:00

RECOMMENDATIONS FOR FLUID INTAKE

- Drink cool (40 degrees F) water. This is the best drink to sustain performance. Fluid also comes from juice, milk, soup, and other beverages.

- Do not drink coffee, tea, and soft drinks even though they provide fluids. The caffeine in them acts as a diuretic which can increase urine production and fluid loss. Avoid alcohol for the same reason.

- Drink large quantities (20 oz.) of water one or two hours before exercise to promote hyperhydration. This allows time for adequate hydration and urination.

- Drink three to six ounces of fluid every 15 to 30 minutes during exercise.

- Replace fluid sweat losses by monitoring pre-and post-exercise body weights. Drink two cups of fluid for every pound of weight lost.

Source: FM 21-20, Physical Fitness Training, US Department of the Army, p. 6-5, 30 September 1992

CHAPTER ELEVEN

ABDOMINAL STRENGTH TRAINING

We see those ads and commercials all the time offering you the opportunity to get your very own six-pack abs just by buying and using this gadget or that gadget or this or that supplement, and mostly within a very brief period of time ranging from 24 hours to 3 months. These gadgets are predominantly and purportedly focusing on the abdominal region and promise that you, too, will lose inches of fat off of your waist, combined with proper diet. Do they work? Will you end up with visible, defined, washboard abs by focusing on exercising your abdominal region? No! It's a myth that any exercise focused on a specific body part will result in the loss of body fat in that specific area. For more details on exercise and diet fairy tales, see the chapter on myths.

Please keep in mind that it is not necessarily a healthy state to have the level of body fat to see clearly defined abs. Just remember that your body also needs body fat. Not enough body fat and too much body fat are both unhealthy states. See the chapter on "Fitness Goals and Progress Measurement" for calculation of your BMI or Body Mass Index.

With these abdominal region exercises below, you will achieve excellent abdominal strength and will also strengthen the surrounding muscles as well, such as lower abs, obliques, hips, thighs and hip flexors. Your cost? Well, the cost of this book. Of course, the real investment is planning and executing your own fitness program as if you were commanding a military operation and your life and the lives of others depended upon it. Guess what?

Your life and the lives of others, who see you and get inspired to do the same, do depend upon the implementation of a consistent exercise and proper eating program.

Let's get started on the road to that six-pack that you so desire and begin with crunches

CRUNCHES

Keep in mind that there are really 1,001 ways to perform this and other body weight exercises. Here's how we will perform the crunch. Get on your back. Take your hands and clasp them behind your head, bend your knees and bring your heels close to your butt. Lift those shoulders up off the ground or floor and lower them again. Start off with 10 to 20 reps per set and work your way up to 50 to 100 or more per set. This is just a slight motion. Concentrate on contracting those abs. Do enough of these and you will notice that the crunch can really work those abs. The motion should be smooth without going too fast.

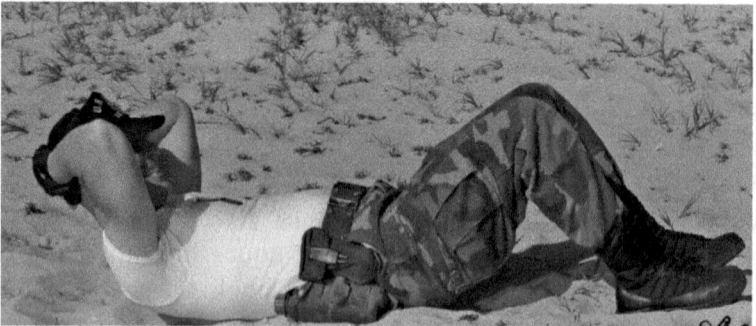

CRUNCHES WITH LEG RAISED AND EXTENDED

Now we're going to vary the crunch by doing crunches with one leg extended off of the ground. Start out with the right leg extended six inches off of the ground and hands still clasped behind your head. We'll practice a set of 30 reps on each leg. Here's how. Perform 10 crunches with the leg six inches off of the ground, then 10 with the leg half way up, then 10 with the leg reaching for the sky. Now switch off and do the same with the left leg or simply switch legs between each set of 10 reps with each leg.

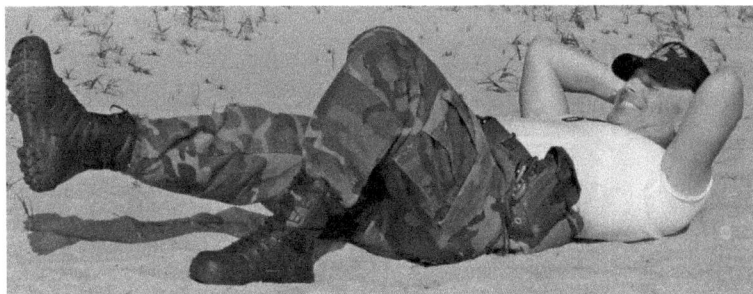

FLUTTER KICKS

You're still on your back with arms extended on the sides of your body and palms facing down to stabilize the lower back and your head raised. Raise up both of your legs in a staggered position (one leg is higher than the other) with a slight bend in the knees. This is a four count exercise. With each count you will simply switch the leg positions which makes it look like a scissor move, not a bicycle pedaling. This is your leg movement for the count: ONE, scissor move; TWO, scissor move; THREE, scissor move; FOUR, scissor move. Here's how you count the reps: One, two, three, ONE; one, two, three, TWO; one, two, three, THREE, one, two, three, FOUR; one, two, three, FIVE. Do five to ten reps per set with multiple sets and very brief rests between sets.

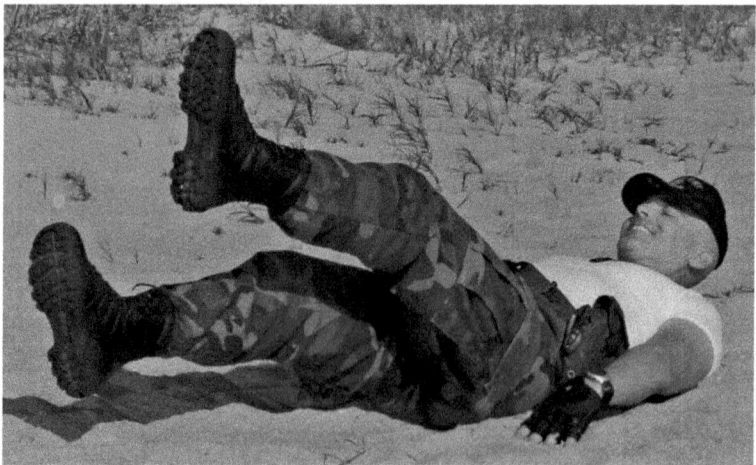

SIT-UPS

Don't you think about getting up! We're not done, yet. Let's get them all done. The next one is a little more advanced. The next exercise is the sit-up. This exercise is one of the events in the Army Physical Fitness Test. If you're not used to doing a sit-up, those muscles will need some developing. Your motion should be smooth, no jerking your body up. If you can't go all the way up, start out by going as far as you can. You're on your back with hands clasped behind your head and feet a little less than shoulder width apart with bent knees and feet on the ground. Curl your body up to the point where you have brought your body out of the range of exertion. When you're out of the range of exertion and it becomes easy, then lower it back down in the starting position with the same smooth motion. That's one repetition. Perform 10 to 50 reps per set. If you are having difficulties, use a slow count until you develop those muscles.

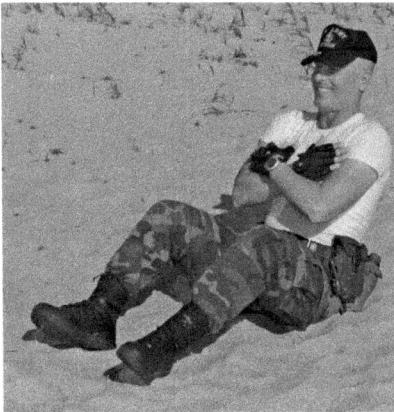

ALTERNATING ELBOW CRUNCH

Here's another great abdominal exercise. We'll call it the alternating elbow crunch. You're on your back. Your hands are clasped behind your head. Your left leg is bent. Cross your right leg over your left knee. Take your left elbow and reach for your right knee and back down. That is one rep. Use a smooth motion. Don't be concerned if you can't reach your leg with your elbow. Do the best you can. Remember, by performing the exercise you are working those muscles! Now switch off by crossing your left leg over your right knee, reach for your knee with your right elbow and do it again.

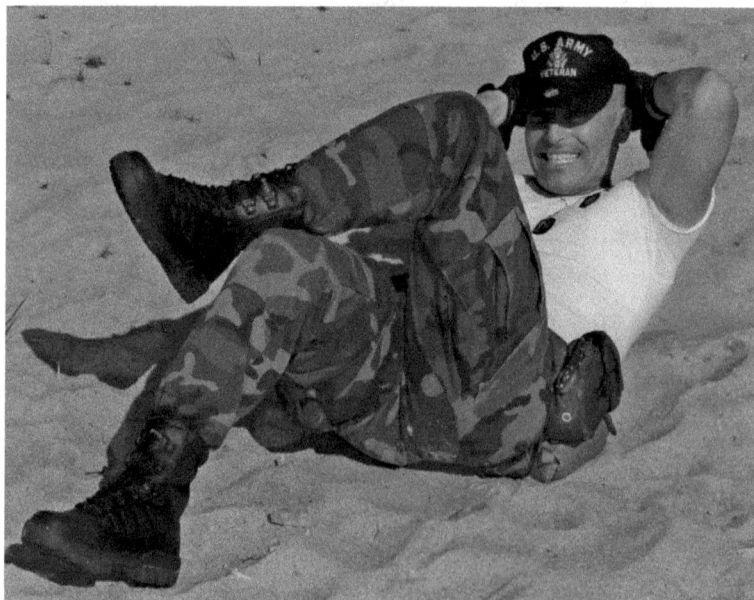

Overview Of Abdominal Exercises

Exercises not found in this book, can be found in my book, *Change Made Easy - Your Basic Training Orders to Excellent Physical and Mental Health.*

Six-pack Abs Workout Guide Reps			
	Beginner	**Intermediate**	**Advanced**
Crunches	10 - 50	50 - 120	120 - 300
Rapid Fire Crunches	10 - 30	30 - 60	60 - 150
Crunches with Leg Raised	10 - 60	60 - 120	120 - 320
4-count Leg Levers	0 - 10	10 - 20	20 - 40
Flutter Kicks	3 - 10	10 - 30	30 - 60
Sit-ups, reps	0 - 10	10 - 40	40 - 100
Reach for the toes!	10 - 40	40 - 60	60 - 100
Alternating Elbow Crunch-up	5 - 10	10 - 30	30 - 60
Atomic Sit-ups	5 - 10	10 - 30	30 - 60

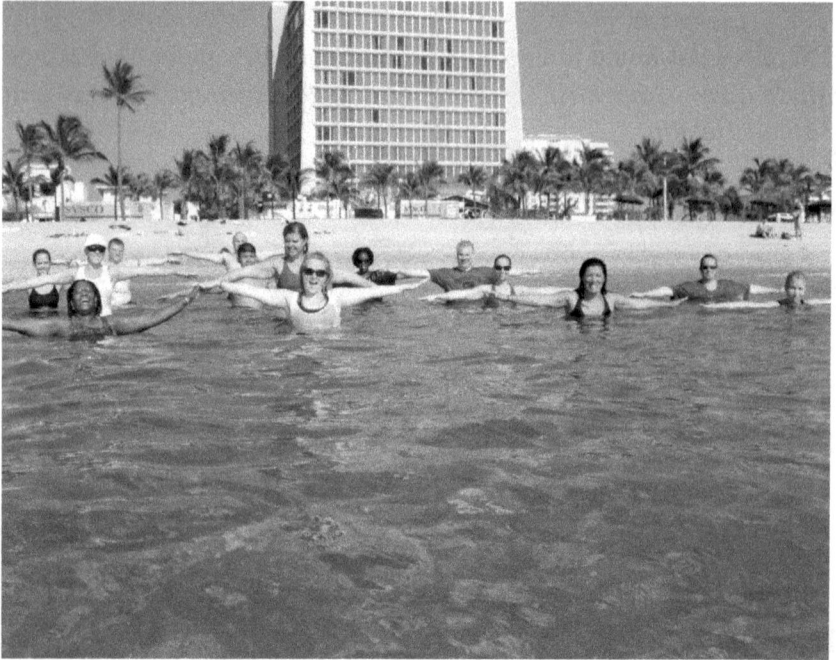

We also take the workouts into the water.

During one of our Saturday Beach Boot Camp classes on Fort Lauderdale Beach in South Florida we took the workout into the ocean. It was very hot that day and a great cool down. Look at the smiles on the faces of these recruits! More photos at www.beachbootcamp.net.

YOUR M.O.V.E. TOOLBOX

HOW TO USE YOUR M.O.V.E. TOOLBOX

Read Before Beginning Your Workout and Weight Loss Plan

Before you embark on your Ten Week Workout Plan, read these instructions carefully, apply them and get moving with *M.O.V.E It to Lose It - Twenty Pounds in Ten Weeks.*

1. Complete the **Physical Activity Readiness-Questionnaire** (PAR-Q). Depending on the results, you may be ready to start your ten week workout.
2. Decide on how much weight you want to lose (up to twenty pounds) in ten weeks and use the appropriate **1,200 or 1,600 calorie sample menu**s as a guide.
3. Complete the **Contract For Change of Lifestyle Habit**.
4. Take **body measurements** as described in Chapter Four, Fitness Goals and Progress Measurement.
5. Photocopy the **Serving Size Card** and laminate and place it in your wallet. Keep this card with you to remind you about proper portion sizes.
6. Familiarize yourself with portion sizes, calories and how many calories you burn with the **Calorie Burn Charts**, **List of Calories in Foods** and the sample **1,200 and 1,600 Calorie Weight-loss Menus** as well as **MyPyramid Food and Calorie Needs Charts**.
7. Photocopy the **Food Diary** and make fourteen copies to track your eating habits for two weeks. Make adjustments where needed. Reduction of quantity and portion sizes are primary ways to lose weight.
8. Photocopy and enlarge the **Workout Log** to track your progress.
9. Get started with your **Ten Week Workout Plan.** Apply these tips and you will maximize your success.
   o Take it one step at a time.
   o Perfect exercise form is not important from a health stand-point. Movement is important. Not quitting is important. Most exercises can be safely modified. If you get too

fatigued, modify the exercise first, then stop, if necessary. Always listen to your body.

○ **Fatigue** is your best friend. If you reach the point of fatigue, that means you're making progress. You must meet my friend fatigue before you can meet my friend progress. Fatigue is the gatekeeper to progress. Never ever apologize for getting fatigued.

○ Your first **fitness test** will be *week 4* of your ten week workout plan. See *Chapter Four, Fitness Goals and Progress Measurement.* Your fitness test is made up of push-ups, crunches and a 1 mile run/walk. See Chapter Four on how to score and conduct your fitness test.

○ If you have been cleared by your physician, you may take a fitness test before starting *week 1.*

○ **Cardio** is your highest fitness priority, not strength and not flexibility.

○ Your goal is to **exercise at least 60 minutes a day**. If you can only do less, then by all means do what you can.

○ Pick the appropriate level of **resistance band** to use (see Chapter Seven - Resistance Band Strength Training). The bands described are from the company SPRI and can be ordered online at **www.spriproducts.com** or at www.amazon.com. If you get too fatigued while using a resistance band, simply do a partial repetition until you complete all reps. The color of a resistance band will impact the workout. Sometimes you will need to switch off, depending on exercises and focus of your training. For example, if you combine heavy cardio with your strength training, you will be more fatigued and may then use a lower level of resistance band to complete the reps.

○ **A set is one sequence.** When Monday, Week 1 of the Ten Week Workout Plan states 2 sets each, that means push-ups, upright row, shoulder press, dips and bicep curls. One set is when you go through the whole sequence of exercises once.

○ **Mix up your workout** to make it more interesting and fun. For example, you may mix your run, walk or jog with your strength training. Stop along the way to complete an exercise and then move on. Keep track of your sets and exercises to make sure you complete them all during your workout session. This is a great way to improve your cardio and your muscular endurance.

○ **Modify your exercises where necessary.** If the number of sets are too many for you to complete, reduce the total number of sets. For example, instead of doing four sets, you modify it to just two.

○ Remember the **WHY** of your exercise program. Your mission is to improve the quality of life and maximize your health. Better health means less illnesses, more energy and a stronger immune system.

A

TEN WEEK

WORKOUT PLAN

FAT AND CALORIE BURNER

WORKOUT - Week 1

MONDAY	TUESDAY	WEDNESDAY
Cardio Walk/jog 15 min. Brief stretch	**Cardio** Walk/jog 15 min. Brief stretch	**Cardio** Walk/jog 15 min. Brief stretch
Upper Body 2 sets each: Push-ups 5 Upright row 10 Shoulder Pr. 5 Dips 10 Bicep Curls 10	**Upper Body** 2 sets each: Push-ups 5 Upright row 10 Shoulder Pr. 5 Dips 10 Bicep Curls 10	**Upper Body** 2 sets each: Push-ups 5 Upright row 10 Shoulder Pr. 5 Dips 10 Bicep Curls 10
Lower Body 2 sets each: Squats 20 Stand.Lunges 20 Dirty Dogs 10 Stand.Crunch 20	**Lower Body** 2 sets each: Squats 20 Stand.Lunges 20 Dirty Dogs 10 Stand.Crunch 20	**Lower Body** 2 sets each: Squats 20 Stand.Lunges 20 Dirty Dogs 10 Stand.Crunch 20
Abs 2 sets each: Crunches 50 4-ct. Leg. Lev. 5 Flutter kicks 5	**Abs** 2 sets each: Crunches 50 4-ct. Leg. Lev. 5 Flutter kicks 5	**Abs** 2 sets each: Crunches 50 4-ct. Leg. Lev. 5 Flutter kicks 5
Stretch 3 min. Upper body Lower body	**Stretch** 3 min. Upper body Lower body	**Stretch** 3 min. Upper body Lower body

WORKOUT - Week 1

THURSDAY	FRIDAY	SATURDAY
Cardio Walk/jog 15 min. Brief stretch	**Cardio** Walk/jog 15 min. Brief stretch	**Cardio** Walk/jog 25 min. Brief stretch
Upper Body 2 sets each: Push-ups 5 Upright row 10 Shoulder Pr. 5 Dips 10 Bicep Curls 10	**Upper Body** 2 sets each: Push-ups 5 Upright row 10 Shoulder Pr. 5 Dips 10 Bicep Curls 10	**Upper Body** 2 sets each: Push-ups 5 Upright row 10 Shoulder Pr. 5 Dips 10 Bicep Curls 10
Lower Body 2 sets each: Squats 20 Stand.Lunges 20 Dirty Dogs 10 Stand.Crunch 20	**Lower Body** 2 sets each: Squats 20 Stand.Lunges 20 Dirty Dogs 10 Stand.Crunch 20	**Lower Body** 2 sets each: Squats 20 Stand.Lunges 20 Dirty Dogs 10 Stand.Crunch 20
Abs 2 sets each: Crunches 50 4-ct. Leg. Lev. 5 Flutter kicks 5	**Abs** 2 sets each: Crunches 50 4-ct. Leg. Lev. 5 Flutter kicks 5	**Abs** 2 sets each: Crunches 50 4-ct. Leg. Lev. 5 Flutter kicks 5
Stretch 3 min. Upper body Lower body	**Stretch** 3 min. Upper body Lower body	**Stretch** 3 min. Upper body Lower body

WORKOUT - Week 2

MONDAY	TUESDAY	WEDNESDAY
Cardio Walk/jog 20 min. Brief stretch	**Cardio** Walk/jog 20 min. Brief stretch	**Cardio** Walk/jog 20 min. Brief stretch
Upper Body 3 sets each: Push-ups 8 Upright row 15 Shoulder Pr. 8 Dips 10 Bicep Curls 10	**Upper Body** 2 sets each: Push-ups 8 Upright row 15 Shoulder Pr. 8 Dips 10 Bicep Curls 10	**Upper Body** 2 sets each: Push-ups 8 Upright row 15 Shoulder Pr. 8 Dips 10 Bicep Curls 10
Lower Body 3 sets each: Squats 30 Stand.Lunges 20 Dirty Dogs 15 Stand.Crunch 30	**Lower Body** 2 sets each: Squats 30 Stand.Lunges 20 Dirty Dogs 15 Stand.Crunch 30	**Lower Body** 2 sets each: Squats 30 Stand.Lunges 20 Dirty Dogs 15 Stand.Crunch 30
Abs 3 sets each: Crunches 50 4-ct. Leg. Lev. 5 Flutter kicks 5 Reach for toes 10	**Abs** 2 sets each: Crunches 50 4-ct. Leg. Lev. 5 Flutter kicks 5 Reach for toes 10	**Abs** 2 sets each: Crunches 50 4-ct. Leg. Lev. 5 Flutter kicks 5 Reach for toes 10
Stretch 3 min. Upper body Lower body	**Stretch** 3 min. Upper body Lower body	**Stretch** 3 min. Upper body Lower body

WORKOUT - Week 2

THURSDAY	FRIDAY	SATURDAY
Cardio Walk/jog 20 min. Brief stretch	**Cardio** Walk/jog 20 min. Brief stretch	**Cardio** Walk/jog 35 min. Brief stretch
Upper Body 2 sets each: Push-ups 8 Upright row 15 Shoulder Pr. 8 Dips 10 Bicep Curls 10	**Upper Body** 2 sets each: Push-ups 8 Upright row 15 Shoulder Pr. 8 Dips 10 Bicep Curls 10	**Upper Body** 2 sets each: Push-ups 5 Upright row 15 Shoulder Pr. 8 Dips 10 Bicep Curls 10
Lower Body 2 sets each: Squats 40 Stand.Lunges 30 Dirty Dogs 30 Stand.Crunch 40	**Lower Body** 2 sets each: Squats 40 Stand.Lunges 30 Dirty Dogs 30 Stand.Crunch 40	**Lower Body** 2 sets each: Squats 30 Stand.Lunges 20 Dirty Dogs 20 Stand.Crunch 30
Abs 2 sets each: Crunches 50 4-ct. Leg. Lev. 5 Flutter kicks 5 Reach for toes 20	**Abs** 2 sets each: Crunches 50 4-ct. Leg. Lev. 5 Flutter kicks 5 Reach for toes 20	**Abs** 2 sets each: Crunches 50 4-ct. Leg. Lev. 5 Flutter kicks 5 Reach for toes 20
Stretch 3 min. Upper body Lower body	**Stretch** 3 min. Upper body Lower body	**Stretch** 3 min. Upper body Lower body

WORKOUT - Week 3

MONDAY	TUESDAY	WEDNESDAY
Cardio	**Cardio**	**Cardio**
Walk/jog 35 min.	Walk/jog 35 min.	Walk/jog 35 min.
Brief stretch	Brief stretch	Brief stretch
Upper Body	**Upper Body**	**Upper Body**
3 sets each:	2 sets each:	2 sets each:
Push-ups 10	Push-ups 15	Push-ups 10
Upright row 20	Upright row 30	Upright row 20
Shoulder Pr. 10	Shoulder Pr. 15	Shoulder Pr. 10
Dips 10	Dips 30	Dips 10
Bicep Curls 10	Bicep Curls 20	Bicep Curls 10
Lower Body	**Lower Body**	**Lower Body**
2 sets each:	2 sets each:	2 sets each:
Squats 50	Squats 20	Squats 50
Stand.Lunges 40	Stand.Lunges 20	Stand.Lunges 40
Dirty Dogs 40	Dirty Dogs 20	Dirty Dogs 40
Stand.Crunch 50	Stand.Crunch 20	Stand.Crunch 20
Abs	**Abs**	**Abs**
2 sets each:	2 sets each:	2 sets each:
Crunches 50	Crunches 50	Crunches 50
4-ct. Leg. Lev. 5	4-ct. Leg. Lev. 5	4-ct. Leg. Lev. 5
Flutter kicks 5	Flutter kicks 5	Flutter kicks 5
Reach for toes 20	Reach for toes 20	Reach for toes 20
Stretch	**Stretch**	**Stretch**
3 min.	3 min.	3 min.
Upper body	Upper body	Upper body
Lower body	Lower body	Lower body

WORKOUT - Week 3

THURSDAY	FRIDAY	SATURDAY
Cardio Walk/jog 35 min. Brief stretch	**Cardio** Walk/jog 35 min. Brief stretch	**Cardio** Walk/jog 35 min. Brief stretch
Upper Body 2 sets each: Push-ups 15 Upright row 30 Shoulder Pr. 15 Dips 30 Bicep Curls 30	**Upper Body** 4 sets each: Push-ups 5 Upright row 10 Shoulder Pr. 5 Dips 10 Bicep Curls 10	**Upper Body** 2 sets each: Push-ups 15 Upright row 30 Shoulder Pr. 15 Dips 30 Bicep Curls 30
Lower Body 2 sets each: Squats 20 Stand.Lunges 20 Dirty Dogs 20 Stand.Crunch 20	**Lower Body** 2 sets each: Squats 50 Stand.Lunges 40 Dirty Dogs 40 Stand.Crunch 50	**Lower Body** 3 sets each: Squats 20 Stand.Lunges 20 Dirty Dogs 10 Stand.Crunch 20
Abs 2 sets each: Crunches 50 4-ct. Leg. Lev. 5 Flutter kicks 5 Reach for toes 20	**Abs** 2 sets each: Crunches 50 4-ct. Leg. Lev. 5 Flutter kicks 5 Reach for toes 20	**Abs** 2 sets each: Crunches 50 4-ct. Leg. Lev. 5 Flutter kicks 5 Reach for toes 20
Stretch 3 min. Upper body Lower body	**Stretch** 3 min. Upper body Lower body	**Stretch** 3 min. Upper body Lower body

WORKOUT - Test Week 4

MONDAY	TUESDAY	WEDNESDAY
Cardio Walk/jog 35 min. Brief stretch Note: If you can jog, do not walk.	**Cardio** Walk/jog 50 min. Brief stretch Note: If you can jog, do not walk.	**Cardio** Walk/jog 40 min. Brief stretch Note: If you can jog, do not walk.
Upper Body 3 sets each: Push-ups 10 Upright row 20 Shoulder Pr. 10 Dips 20 Bicep Curls 15	**Upper Body** 1 set each: Push-ups 5 Upright row 10 Shoulder Pr. 5 Dips 10 Bicep Curls 10	**Upper Body** 2 sets each: Push-ups 10 Upright row 10 Shoulder Pr. 10 Dips 10 Bicep Curls 10
Lower Body 2 sets each: Squats 20 Stand.Lunges 20 Dirty Dogs 20 Stand.Crunch 20	**Lower Body** 1 set each: Squats 20 Stand.Lunges 20 Dirty Dogs 10 Stand.Crunch 20	**Lower Body** 2 sets each: Squats 20 Stand.Lunges 20 Dirty Dogs 20 Stand.Crunch 20
Abs 2 sets each: Crunches 50 4-ct. Leg. Lev. 8 Flutter kicks 8 Reach for toes 10	**Abs** 1 set each: Crunches 50 4-ct. Leg. Lev. 5 Flutter kicks 5 Reach for toes 10	**Abs** 2 sets each: Crunches 50 4-ct. Leg. Lev. 5 Flutter kicks 5 Reach for toes 10
Stretch 3 min. Upper body Lower body	**Stretch** 3 min. Upper body Lower body	**Stretch** 3 min. Upper body Lower body

WORKOUT - Test Week 4

THURSDAY	FRIDAY	SATURDAY
Cardio Walk/jog 30 min. Brief stretch Note: If you can jog, do not walk.	**Cardio** Walk/jog 30 min. Brief stretch Note: If you can jog, do not walk.	**M.O.V.E. Fitness Test** - Push-ups (2 min.) - Crunches (2 min.) - 1-mile run for time - Body measurements NOTE: See chapter on goals and progress measurement for more detail.
Upper Body 2 sets each: Push-ups 5 Upright row 10 Shoulder Pr. 5 Dips 10 Bicep Curls 10	**Upper Body** 1 set each: Push-ups 5 Upright row 10 Shoulder Pr. 5 Dips 10 Bicep Curls 10	**Upper Body** 1 set each: Push-ups 5 Upright row 10 Shoulder Pr. 5 Dips 10 Bicep Curls 10
Lower Body 2 sets each: Squats 20 Stand.Lunges 20 Dirty Dogs 10 Stand.Crunch 20	**Lower Body** 1 set each: Squats 20 Stand.Lunges 20 Dirty Dogs 10 Stand.Crunch 20	**Lower Body** 1 set each: Squats 20 Stand.Lunges 10 Dirty Dogs 10 Stand.Crunch 10
Abs 2 sets each: Crunches 50 4-ct. Leg. Lev. 5 Flutter kicks 5 Reach for toes 10	**Abs** 1 set each: Crunches 50 4-ct. Leg. Lev. 5 Flutter kicks 5 Reach for toes 10	**Abs** 1 set each: Crunches 50 4-ct. Leg. Lev. 5 Flutter kicks 5 Reach for toes 10
Stretch 3 min. Upper body Lower body	**Stretch** 3 min. Upper body Lower body	**Stretch** 3 min. Upper body Lower body

WORKOUT - Week 5

MONDAY	TUESDAY	WEDNESDAY
Cardio Walk/jog 30 min. Brief stretch Note: If you can jog, do not walk.	**Cardio** Walk/jog 50 min. Brief stretch Note: If you can jog, do not walk. **Intervals**: 5 sets of 50 to 100 yards each	**Cardio** Walk/jog 30 min. Brief stretch Note: If you can jog, do not walk.
Upper Body 3 sets each: Push-ups 15 Upright row 30 Shoulder Pr. 10 Dips 20 Bicep Curls 20	**Upper Body** 1 set each: Push-ups 20 Upright row 30 Shoulder Pr. 20 Dips 40 Bicep Curls 40	**Upper Body** 2 sets each: Push-ups 20 Upright row 40 Shoulder Pr. 15 Dips 30 Bicep Curls 30
Lower Body 2 sets each:A1 Squats 40 Stand.Lunges 30 Dirty Dogs 30 Stand.Crunch 40	**Lower Body** 1 set each: Squats 50 Stand.Lunges 40 Dirty Dogs 50 Stand.Crunch 50	**Lower Body** 2 sets each: Squats 50 Stand.Lunges 40 Dirty Dogs 40 Stand.Crunch 40
Abs 2 sets each: Crunches 50 4-ct. Leg. Lev. 10 Flutter kicks 10 Reach for toes 40	**Abs** 1 set each: Crunches 100 4-ct. Leg. Lev. 10 Flutter kicks 10 Reach for toes 40	**Abs** 2 sets each: Crunches 50 4-ct. Leg. Lev. 10 Flutter kicks 10 Reach for toes 40
Stretch 3 min. Upper body Lower body	**Stretch** 3 min. Upper body Lower body	**Stretch** 3 min. Upper body Lower body

WORKOUT - Week 5

THURSDAY	FRIDAY	SATURDAY
Cardio Walk/jog 50 min. Brief stretch Note: If you can jog, do not walk. **Intervals**: 5 sets of 50 to 100 yards each	**Cardio** Walk/jog 30 min. Brief stretch Note: If you can jog, do not walk.	**Cardio** Walk/jog 50 min. Brief stretch Note: If you can jog, do not walk. **Intervals**: 5 sets of 50 to 100 yards each
Upper Body 1 set each: Push-ups 20 Upright row 30 Shoulder Pr. 20 Dips 40 Bicep Curls 40	**Upper Body** 3 sets each: Push-ups 15 Upright row 30 Shoulder Pr. 10 Dips 20 Bicep Curls 20	**Upper Body** 3 sets each: Push-ups 15 Upright row 30 Shoulder Pr. 10 Dips 20 Bicep Curls 20
Lower Body 1 set each: Squats 50 Stand.Lunges 40 Dirty Dogs 50 Stand.Crunch 50	**Lower Body** 3 sets each: Squats 40 Stand.Lunges 30 Dirty Dogs 30 Stand.Crunch 40	**Lower Body** 2 sets each: Squats 40 Stand.Lunges 30 Dirty Dogs 30 Stand.Crunch 50
Abs 1 set each: Crunches 100 4-ct. Leg. Lev. 10 Flutter kicks 10 Reach for toes 40	**Abs** 2 sets each: Crunches 50 4-ct. Leg. Lev. 10 Flutter kicks 10 Reach for toes 40	**Abs** 2 sets each: Crunches 50 4-ct. Leg. Lev. 10 Flutter kicks 10 Reach for toes 40
Stretch 3 min. Upper body Lower body	**Stretch** 3 min. Upper body Lower body	**Stretch** 3 min. Upper body Lower body

WORKOUT - Week 6

MONDAY	TUESDAY	WEDNESDAY
Cardio	**Cardio**	**Cardio**
Walk/jog 50 min.	Walk/jog 30 min.	Walk/jog 50 min.
Brief stretch	Brief stretch	Brief stretch
Note: If you can jog, do not walk.	Note: If you can jog, do not walk.	Note: If you can jog, do not walk.
Intervals: 5 sets of 50 to 100 yards each		
Upper Body	**Upper Body**	**Upper Body**
1 set each:	3 sets each:	1 set each:
Push-ups 30	Push-ups 20	Push-ups 30
Upright row 40	Upright row 30	Upright row 40
Shoulder Pr. 20	Shoulder Pr. 10	Shoulder Pr. 20
Dips 40	Dips 30	Dips 40
Bicep Curls 40	Bicep Curls 10	Bicep Curls 30
Lower Body	**Lower Body**	**Lower Body**
1 set each:	3 sets each:	1 set each:
Squats 50	Squats 50	Squats 50
Stand.Lunges 40	Stand.Lunges 30	Stand.Lunges 40
Dirty Dogs 50	Dirty Dogs 40	Dirty Dogs 50
Stand.Crunch 50	Stand.Crunch 40	Stand.Crunch 50
Abs	**Abs**	**Abs**
1 set each:	2 sets each:	1 set each:
Crunches 100	Crunches 50	Crunches 100
4-ct. Leg. Lev. 10	4-ct. Leg. Lev. 10	4-ct. Leg. Lev. 10
Flutter kicks 10	Flutter kicks 10	Flutter kicks 10
Reach for toes 40	Reach for toes 40	Reach for toes 40
Stretch	**Stretch**	**Stretch**
3 min.	3 min.	3 min.
Upper body	Upper body	Upper body
Lower body	Lower body	Lower body

WORKOUT - Week 6

THURSDAY	FRIDAY	SATURDAY
Cardio	**Cardio**	**Cardio**
Walk/jog 30 min.	Walk/jog 50 min.	Walk/jog 30 min.
Brief stretch	Brief stretch	Brief stretch
Note: If you can jog, do not walk.	Note: If you can jog, do not walk.	Note: If you can jog, do not walk.
	Intervals: 5 sets of 50 to 100 yards each	
Upper Body	**Upper Body**	**Upper Body**
5 sets each:	1 set each:	4 sets each:
Push-ups 10	Push-ups 30	Push-ups 10
Upright row 15	Upright row 40	Upright row 15
Shoulder Pr. 10	Shoulder Pr. 20	Shoulder Pr. 10
Dips 10	Dips 40	Dips 10
Bicep Curls 10	Bicep Curls 40	Bicep Curls 10
Lower Body	**Lower Body**	**Lower Body**
4 sets each:	1 set each:	3 sets each:
Squats 30	Squats 50	Squats 30
Stand.Lunges 20	Stand.Lunges 40	Stand.Lunges 20
Dirty Dogs 20	Dirty Dogs 50	Dirty Dogs 20
Stand.Crunch 20	Stand.Crunch 50	Stand.Crunch 30
Abs	**Abs**	**Abs**
2 sets each:	1 set each:	2 sets each:
Crunches 50	Crunches 50	Crunches 50
4-ct. Leg. Lev. 10	4-ct. Leg. Lev. 10	4-ct. Leg. Lev. 10
Flutter kicks 10	Flutter kicks 10	Flutter kicks 10
Reach for toes 40	Reach for toes 40	Reach for toes 40
Stretch	**Stretch**	**Stretch**
3 min.	3 min.	3 min.
Upper body	Upper body	Upper body
Lower body	Lower body	Lower body

WORKOUT - Week 7

MONDAY	TUESDAY	WEDNESDAY
Cardio Walk/jog 30 min. Brief stretch Note: If you can jog, do not walk.	**Cardio** Walk/jog 50 min. Brief stretch Note: If you can jog, do not walk.	**Cardio** Walk/jog 50 min. Brief stretch Note: If you can jog, do not walk. **Intervals**: 5 sets of 50 to 100 yards each
Upper Body 4 sets each: Push-ups 10 Upright row 15 Shoulder Pr. 10 Dips 10 Bicep Curls 10	**Upper Body** 2 sets each: Push-ups 5 Upright row 10 Shoulder Pr. 5 Dips 10 Bicep Curls 10	**Upper Body** 1 set each: Push-ups 40 Upright row 40 Shoulder Pr. 20 Dips 40 Bicep Curls 40
Lower Body 5 sets each: Squats 30 Stand.Lunges 20 Dirty Dogs 20 Stand.Crunch 20	**Lower Body** 2 sets each: Squats 20 Stand.Lunges 20 Dirty Dogs 10 Stand.Crunch 20	**Lower Body** 1 set each: Squats 50 Stand.Lunges 40 Dirty Dogs 30 Stand.Crunch 30
Abs 2 sets each: Crunches 50 4-ct. Leg. Lev. 10 Flutter kicks 10 Reach for toes 40	**Abs** 1 set each: Crunches 50 4-ct. Leg. Lev. 10 Flutter kicks 10 Reach for toes 40	**Abs** 1 set each: Crunches 50 4-ct. Leg. Lev. 10 Flutter kicks 10 Reach for toes 40
Stretch 3 min. Upper body Lower body	**Stretch** 3 min. Upper body Lower body	**Stretch** 3 min. Upper body Lower body

WORKOUT - Week 7

THURSDAY	FRIDAY	SATURDAY
Cardio	**Cardio**	**Cardio**
Walk/jog 40 min.	Walk/jog 30 min.	Walk/jog 50 min.
Brief stretch	Brief stretch	Brief stretch
Note: If you can jog, do not walk.	Note: If you can jog, do not walk.	Note: If you can jog, do not walk.
		Intervals: 5 sets of 50 to 100 yards each
Upper Body	**Upper Body**	**Upper Body**
5 sets each:	3 sets each:	1 set each:
Push-ups 10	Push-ups 20	Push-ups 30
Upright row 15	Upright row 30	Upright row 40
Shoulder Pr. 10	Shoulder Pr. 10	Shoulder Pr. 10
Dips 10	Dips 20	Dips 30
Bicep Curls 10	Bicep Curls 20	Bicep Curls 30
Lower Body	**Lower Body**	**Lower Body**
4 sets each:	2 sets each:	1 set each:
Squats 20	Squats 20	Squats 50
Stand.Lunges 20	Stand.Lunges 20	Stand.Lunges 40
Dirty Dogs 20	Dirty Dogs 10	Dirty Dogs 30
Stand.Crunch 20	Stand.Crunch 20	Stand.Crunch 30
Abs	**Abs**	**Abs**
2 sets each:	2 sets each:	1 set each:
Crunches 50	Crunches 50	Crunches 100
4-ct. Leg. Lev. 10	4-ct. Leg. Lev. 10	4-ct. Leg. Lev. 10
Flutter kicks 10	Flutter kicks 10	Flutter kicks 10
Reach for toes 30	Reach for toes 40	Reach for toes 40
Stretch	**Stretch**	**Stretch**
3 min.	3 min.	3 min.
Upper body	Upper body	Upper body
Lower body	Lower body	Lower body

WORKOUT - Test Week 8

MONDAY	TUESDAY	WEDNESDAY
Cardio Walk/jog 30 min. Brief stretch Note: If you can jog, do not walk.	**Cardio** Walk/jog 30 min. Brief stretch Note: If you can jog, do not walk.	**Cardio** Walk/jog 40 min. Brief stretch Note: If you can jog, do not walk.
Upper Body 5 sets each: Push-ups 10 Upright row 10 Shoulder Pr. 10 Dips 10 Bicep Curls 10	**Upper Body** 4 sets each: Push-ups 10 Upright row 10 Shoulder Pr. 10 Dips 10 Bicep Curls 10	**Upper Body** 3 sets each: Push-ups 10 Upright row 10 Shoulder Pr. 10 Dips 10 Bicep Curls 10
Lower Body 3 sets each: Squats 30 Stand.Lunges 20 Dirty Dogs 20 Stand.Crunch 20	**Lower Body** 2 sets each: Squats 20 Stand.Lunges 20 Dirty Dogs 20 Stand.Crunch 20	**Lower Body** 2 sets each: Squats 30 Stand.Lunges 20 Dirty Dogs 20 Stand.Crunch 20
Abs 2 sets each: Crunches 50 4-ct. Leg. Lev. 10 Flutter kicks 10 Reach for toes 40	**Abs** 2 sets each: Crunches 50 4-ct. Leg. Lev. 10 Flutter kicks 10 Reach for toes 40	**Abs** 2 sets each: Crunches 50 4-ct. Leg. Lev. 10 Flutter kicks 10 Reach for toes 40
Stretch 3 min. Upper body Lower body	**Stretch** 3 min. Upper body Lower body	**Stretch** 3 min. Upper body Lower body

WORKOUT - Test Week 8

THURSDAY	FRIDAY	SATURDAY
Cardio	**Cardio**	**M.O.V.E. Fitness Test**
Walk/jog 40 min.	Walk/jog 30 min.	- Push-ups (2 min.)
Brief stretch	Brief stretch	- Crunches (2 min.)
Note: If you can jog, do	Note: If you can jog, do	- 1-mile run for time
not walk.	not walk.	- Body measurements
		NOTE: See chapter on
		goals and progress mea-
		surement for more detail.
Upper Body	**Upper Body**	**Upper Body**
2 sets each:	1 set each:	1 set each:
Push-ups 20	Push-ups 20	Push-ups 5
Upright row 20	Upright row 30	Upright row 10
Shoulder Pr. 10	Shoulder Pr. 10	Shoulder Pr. 5
Dips 10	Dips 10	Dips 10
Bicep Curls 10	Bicep Curls 20	Bicep Curls 10
Lower Body	**Lower Body**	**Lower Body**
2 sets each:	1 set each:	1 set each:
Squats 30	Squats 50	Squats 20
Stand.Lunges 20	Stand.Lunges 20	Stand.Lunges 10
Dirty Dogs 20	Dirty Dogs 30	Dirty Dogs 10
Stand.Crunch 20	Stand.Crunch 30	Stand.Crunch 10
Abs	**Abs**	**Abs**
2 sets each:	1 set each:	1 set each:
Crunches 50	Crunches 50	Crunches 50
4-ct. Leg. Lev. 10	4-ct. Leg. Lev. 5	4-ct. Leg. Lev. 10
Flutter kicks 10	Flutter kicks 5	Flutter kicks 10
Reach for toes 40	Reach for toes 40	Reach for toes 10
Stretch	**Stretch**	**Stretch**
3 min.	3 min.	3 min.
Upper body	Upper body	Upper body
Lower body	Lower body	Lower body

WORKOUT - Week 9

MONDAY	TUESDAY	WEDNESDAY
Cardio	**Cardio**	**Cardio**
Walk/jog 30 min.	Walk/jog 30 min.	Walk/jog 50 min.
Brief stretch	Brief stretch	Brief stretch
Note: If you can jog, do not walk.	Note: If you can jog, do not walk.	Note: If you can jog, do not walk.
Upper Body	**Upper Body**	**Upper Body**
1 set each:	4 sets each:	1 set each:
Push-ups 30	Push-ups 20	Push-ups 30
Upright row 40	Upright row 20	Upright row 30
Shoulder Pr. 20	Shoulder Pr. 10	Shoulder Pr. 10
Dips 40	Dips 10	Dips 40
Bicep Curls 30	Bicep Curls 10	Bicep Curls 30
Lower Body	**Lower Body**	**Lower Body**
1 set each:	2 sets each:	1 set each:
Squats 100	Squats 50	Squats 50
Stand.Lunges 40	Stand.Lunges 30	Stand.Lunges 30
Dirty Dogs 50	Dirty Dogs 30	Dirty Dogs 30
Stand.Crunch 50	Stand.Crunch 40	Stand.Crunch 30
Abs	**Abs**	**Abs**
1 set each:	2 sets each:	1 set each:
Crunches 100	Crunches 50	Crunches 50
4-ct. Leg. Lev. 10	4-ct. Leg. Lev. 10	4-ct. Leg. Lev. 10
Flutter kicks 10	Flutter kicks 10	Flutter kicks 10
Reach for toes 50	Reach for toes 40	Reach for toes 40
Stretch	**Stretch**	**Stretch**
3 min.	3 min.	3 min.
Upper body	Upper body	Upper body
Lower body	Lower body	Lower body

WORKOUT - Week 9

THURSDAY	FRIDAY	SATURDAY
Cardio Walk/jog 40 min. Brief stretch Note: If you can jog, do not walk.	**Cardio** Walk/jog 50 min. Brief stretch Note: If you can jog, do not walk.	**Cardio** Walk/jog 40 min. Brief stretch Note: If you can jog, do not walk.
Upper Body 1 set each: Upright row 50 Shoulder Pr. 20 Bicep Curls 40	**Upper Body** 1 set each: Push-ups 40 Dips 50	**Upper Body** 1 set each: Push-ups 40 Dips 50
Lower Body 1 set each: Squats 50 Stand.Crunch 50	**Lower Body** 1 set each: Stand.L30 Dirty Dogs 30	**Lower Body** 1 set each: Squats 50 Stand.Crunch 50
Abs 2 sets each: Crunches 50 4-ct. Leg. Lev. 10 Flutter kicks 10 Reach for toes 40	**Abs** 2 sets each: Crunches 50 4-ct. Leg. Lev. 10 Flutter kicks 10 Reach for toes 40	**Abs** 2 sets each: Crunches 50 4-ct. Leg. Lev. 10 Flutter kicks 10 Reach for toes 40
Stretch 3 min. Upper body Lower body	**Stretch** 3 min. Upper body Lower body	**Stretch** 3 min. Upper body Lower body

WORKOUT - Week 10

MONDAY	TUESDAY	WEDNESDAY
Cardio	**Cardio**	**Cardio**
Walk/jog 50 min.	Walk/jog 50 min.	Walk/jog 50 min.
Brief stretch	Brief stretch	Brief stretch
Note: If you can jog, do not walk.	Note: If you can jog, do not walk.	Note: If you can jog, do not walk.
Upper Body	**Upper Body**	**Upper Body**
5 sets each:	4 sets each:	1 set each:
Push-ups 10	Upright row 30	Push-ups 50
Dips 20	Shoulder Pr. 10	Dips 50
	Bicep Curls 20	
Lower Body	**Lower Body**	**Lower Body**
5 sets each:	4 sets each:	1 set each:
Stand.Lunges 20	Squats 50	Squats 100
Dirty Dogs 20		Stand.Crunch 50
Abs	**Abs**	**Abs**
1 set each:	2 sets each:	1 set each:
Crunches 100	Crunches 50	Crunches 100
4-ct. Leg. Lev. 10	4-ct. Leg. Lev. 10	4-ct. Leg. Lev. 10
Flutter kicks 10	Flutter kicks 10	Flutter kicks 10
Reach for toes 40	Reach for toes 40	Reach for toes 40
Stretch	**Stretch**	**Stretch**
3 min.	3 min.	3 min.
Upper body	Upper body	Upper body
Lower body	Lower body	Lower body

WORKOUT - Week 10

THURSDAY	FRIDAY	SATURDAY
Cardio Walk/jog 50 min. Brief stretch Note: If you can jog, do not walk.	**Cardio** Walk/jog 50 min. Brief stretch Note: If you can jog, do not walk.	**Cardio** Walk/jog 50 min. Brief stretch Note: If you can jog, do not walk.
Upper Body 2 sets each: Push-ups 20 Dips 30	**Upper Body** 1 set each: Upright row 40 Shoulder Pr. 20 Bicep Curls 30	**Upper Body** 1 set each: Push-ups 40 Upright row 30 Shoulder Pr. 10 Dips 30 Bicep Curls 30
Lower Body 1 set each: Squats 50 Stand.Lunges 20 Dirty Dogs 30 Stand.Crunch 30	**Lower Body** 1 set each: Squats 50 Stand.Lunges 30 Stand.Crunch 40	**Lower Body** 1 set each: Squats 50 Stand.Lunges 30
Abs 1 set each: Crunches 50 4-ct. Leg. Lev. 10 Flutter kicks 10 Reach for toes 40	**Abs** 1 set each: Crunches 50 4-ct. Leg. Lev. 10 Flutter kicks 10 Reach for toes 40	**Abs** 1 set each: Crunches 50 4-ct. Leg. Lev. 10 Flutter kicks 10 Reach for toes 40
Stretch 3 min. Upper body Lower body	**Stretch** 3 min. Upper body Lower body	**Stretch** 3 min. Upper body Lower body

B

WORKOUT GUIDELINES

All workouts follow the **F.I.T.T. guidelines**. Guidelines are created for:

F. = Frequency of exercise.
I. = Intensity (Very hard, Hard, Moderate, Light, Very Light).
T. = Time (or duration). How long.
T. = Type of exercise (walking, biking, shoulder press, push-ups, etc.)

Note: Always Warm-up for about 10 minutes before actual exercising or stretching (Warm-up light walking, break a light sweat. Warms up the core muscles to prevent injury and maximize muscle performance.)

A. Cardio workouts.

    a. Frequency. 3 to 6 days per week, (7th day light only =active recovery)

    b. Intensity. First 3 weeks light. After 3rd week light to moderate.

    c. Time. At least 15 minutes, preferably 20 to 30 minutes the first 3 weeks. After the 3rd week, 30 to 60 minutes.

    Note: If necessary, breakdown the times, for example, into two parts (example: 20 min. walk in the morning, and then later in the day, 20 min. treadmill).

    d. Type (or Mode). Walk, stationary bike, treadmill or swim.

B. Strength Training (With weight machines, gym)
   a. Frequency. Twice per week.
   b. Intensity. First 6 weeks, 1 set of 12 or greater repetitions per exercise with "low" weights (30 % of 1 RM=30% of maximum amount to fatigue for 1 repetition). Stretch between each exercise performed.
   c. Time. Take your time. Wait 2 minutes or more between sets.
   d. Type (or Mode).
      i. Legs. Leg press and leg extension.
      ii.   **Hips.** Hip flexion and hip extension.
      iii. **Abdominal.** Crunch.
      iv. **Low back.** Back extension. (check with Chiropractor)
      v.   **Torso.** Chest press.
      vi. **Torso.** Shoulder press.

C. Strength Training (With resistance band and body weight exercises = home or gym) (Alternate upper and lower body exercises and use crunches to "fill in the gaps since you don't have that many lower body exercises).
   a. Frequency. Twice per week.
   b. Intensity. Make the effort to perform at least 15 reps and not less then 10 reps with resistance band per exercise. A little struggle is okay. The effort should be light to moderate for the first 4 weeks, which means that you may have to adjust the repetitions. Stretch between each exercise performed. Extra sets of crunches are okay.
   c. Time. Take your time. Wait 2 minutes or more between sets. "Listen" to your body while working out.

d. Type (or Mode). (RB = Resistance Band)
   i. Legs. Squats. (Do two sets of these)

     ii.   Hips.
         Side Lying Abductors and squats (one set each)
     iii. Abdominal. Crunch. (Use crunches as a "rest" exercise)
     iv. Low back. Back extension (check with Chiropractor)
     v.   Torso. Upright row. (RB)
     vi. Torso. Biceps curl. (RB)
     vii. Torso. Shoulder press. (RB)
     viii. Torso. Front raise. (RB)
     ix. Torso. Side lateral raise (RB)
     x.   Torso. Dips. (Bench or chair).
     xi. Torso. One arm triceps work with arm behind head and ball of foot on band while in standing position (about six inches from one end, raise band up behind your head). Do both arms. (RB)
     xii. Torso. Push-ups.

NOTE: Do 5 to 10 sets of each exercise. Instead of simply performing all sets at once, alternative between various exercises and pace yourself so that you can continue. Adjust the reps according to how you feel you can do to perform the 5 to 10 sets.

FITT Factors Applied to Physical Conditioning Program

	Cardiorespiratory Endurance	Muscular Strength	Muscular Endurance	Muscular Strength and Muscular Endurance	Flexibility
F Frequency	3-5 times/week	3 times/week	3-5 times/week	3 times/week	Warm-up and Cool-down: Stretch before and after each exercise session Developmental Stretching: To improve flexibility, stretch 2-3 times/week
I Intensity	60-90% HRR*	3-7 RM*	12+ RM	8-12 RM	Tension and slight discomfort, NOT PAIN
T Time	20 minutes or more	The time required to do 3-7 repetitions of each exercise	The time required to do 12+ repetitions of each exercise	The time required to do 8-12 repetitions of each exercise	Warm-up and Cool-down Stretches: 10-15 seconds/stretch Developmental Stretches: 30-60 seconds/stretch
T Type	Running Swimming Cross-Country Skiing Rowing Bicycling Jumping Rope Walking/Hiking Stair Climbing	Free Weights Resistance Machines Partner-Resisted Exercises Body-Weight Exercises (Pushups/Situps/Pullups/Dips, etc.)			Stretching: Static Passive P.N.F.

* HRR = Heart Rate Reserve   * RM = Repetition Maximum

*Source: FM 21-20, Physical Fitness Training, Hqs Dept. Of the Army, p. 1-5,
Figure 1-1*

C

Exercise Chart Overview

Exercise	Beginner	Intermediate	Advanced	Pg
Regular Push-up, reps	2 - 20	20 - 30	30 - 100	86
Regular Dips, reps	5 - 15	15 - 40	40 - 100	87
Leg Extended Dips, reps (each leg)	5 - 10	10 - 20	20 - 40	88
Bicep Curls, reps	5 - 30	30 - 60	60 - 100	93
Upright Row, reps	5 - 40	40 - 60	60 - 100	94
Shoulder Press, reps	3 - 10	10 - 15	15 - 40	95
Standing Row, reps	10 - 40	40 - 70	70 - 100	96
Standing Triceps Push, reps	5 - 10	10 - 20	20 - 30	97
Squats, reps	20 - 40	40 - 100	100 - 200	102
Dirty Dogs, reps, each leg	5 - 10	10 - 40	40 - 80	104
Leg Thrusts, reps, each leg	5 - 20	20 - 50	50 - 80	105
Alternating Side Leg Raise (Lift)	10 - 15	15 - 30	30 - 70	106
Walking Lunges	10 - 20	20 - 40	40 - 100	103
Jumping Jacks	10 - 30	30 - 50	50 - 100	110
Wind Mills, 4 count	5 - 15	15 - 30	30 - 80	111
Snap Kick, each leg	10 - 30	30 - 60	60 - 100	112
Side Punch Drill, 4 count	10 - 30	30 - 60	60 - 100	113
Toe Raisers, 4 count	20 - 40	40 - 70	70 - 100	114
Run 1 Mile	11:00-18:00	8:00-11:00	5:00-8:00	
Run 2 Miles	16:00-30:00	14:00-16:00	10:00-14:00	
Crunches	10 - 50	50 - 120	120 - 300	124
Crunches with Leg Raised	10 - 60	60 - 120	120 - 320	125
Flutter Kicks	3 - 10	10 - 30	30 - 60	126
Alternating Elbow Crunch-up	5 - 10	10 - 30	30 - 60	128

Nine ways of thinking that could lead to your demise:

1. Adopt a pill popping mentality.
2. Adopt a Can't-do-anything-to-change-it mentality.
3. Adopt a closed mind.
4. Failed to ask, "Am I doing all that's reasonably possible?"
5. Adopt a disregard cause-and-effect mentality.
6. Adopt a philosophy of sedentary lifestyle.
7. Adopt a disregard-what-is-most-important mentality.
8. Eat predominantly refined foods.
9. Think that BMI stands for Big Mac Injection.

EXERCISE CHART FOR MUSCULAR STRENGTH AND ENDURANCE

EXERCISES	LOWER LEGS	UPPER LEGS	WAIST	CHEST	UPPER ARMS	LOWER ARMS	SHOULDERS	BACK
Partner-Resisted Exercises								
Split-Squat		x						
Single-Leg Squat		x						
Leg Extension		x						
Leg Curl		x						
Heel Raise	x							
Toe Raise	x							
Push-Up				x	x			
Seated Row					x			x
Overhead Press					x		x	
Pull-Down					x			x
Shrug							x	
Triceps Extension					x			
Biceps Curl					x			
Abdominal Twist			x					
Abdominal Curl			x					
Abdominal Crunch			x					
Exercises with Equipment (Barbell/Dumbbell)								
Squat		x						
Heel Raise	x							
Bench Press				x	x			
Bent-Over Row					x			x
Overhead Press					x		x	
Shrug							x	
Triceps Extension					x			
Biceps Curl					x			
Wrist Curl						x		
Bent-Leg Dead Lift		x					x	x
Exercises with an Exercise Machine								
Leg Press		x						
Leg Extension		x						
Leg Curl		x						
Heel Raise	x							
Toe Raise	x							
Bench Press				x	x			
Seated Row					x			x
Lat Pull-Down					x			x
Shrug							x	
Parallel Bar Dip				x	x			
Chin-up					x			x
Triceps Extension					x			
Biceps Curl					x			
Back Extension								x
Sit-Up			x					
Incline Sit-Up			x					
Abdominal Twist			x					
Abdominal Crunch			x					

Figure 3-5

Source: FM 21-20, Physical Fitness Training, HQ Dept. Of the Army, p. 3-8, Figure 3-5

DAILY FOOD GUIDE

Eat a variety of foods from each food group. Most people should have the minimum number of servings; others need more due to their body size and activity level.

FOOD GROUP	SUGGESTED NUMBER OF SERVINGS	SUGGESTED SIZE OF SERVINGS
Vegetables (Include dark green, leafy, or deep yellow ones)	3 to 5	1 cup of raw, leafy greens or 1/2 cup of cooked vegetables
Fruits (Include citrus fruits or juices, melons, or berries)	2 to 4	1 medium fruit or 1/2 cup of diced or small fruit or 3/4 cup of juice
Breads, Cereals, Rice, and Pasta (Include whole grain varieties)	6 to 11	1 slice of bread, 1/2 bun or roll, 1/2 cup of cooked cereal, rice or pasta, 1 oz. of ready-to-eat cereal
Milk, Yogurt, and Cheese (Include skim or lowfat varieties)	2 to 3	1 cup of milk or yogurt, 1-1/2 oz. of hard cheese
Meats, Poultry, Fish, Dry Beans or Peas, Eggs, Nuts (Use lean meats and remove skin from poultry)	2 to 3	2 or 3 oz. of cooked meat, fish, or poultry (TOTAL 6 oz/day) 2 eggs, or 1 cup of cooked beans or peas

Source: FM 21-20, Physical Fitness Training, US Department of the Army, p. 6-1, 30 September 1992

D

SAMPLE CIRCUIT FOR CARDIORESPIRATORY ENDURANCE

STATION #1

Stationary Run
30 seconds

STATION #14

All-Fours Run
30 seconds

STATION #2

Push-Up
30 seconds

Do 2-3 complete rotations.

STATION #13

Mule Kicks
30 seconds

STATION #3

Side-Straddle Hop
30 seconds

Stations may be 25-30 meters
apart to allow more running.

STATION #12

Twisting Sit-up
30 seconds

STATION #4

Sit-Up
30 seconds

STATION #11

Steam Engine
30 seconds

STATION #5

Ski Jumps
30 seconds

STATION #10

Knee Bender
30 seconds

STATION #6

Flutter Kicks
30 seconds

STATION #9

Bicycle
30 seconds

STATION #8

Wide-Hand Push-Ups
30 seconds

STATION #7

Bend and Reach
(done slowly)
30 seconds

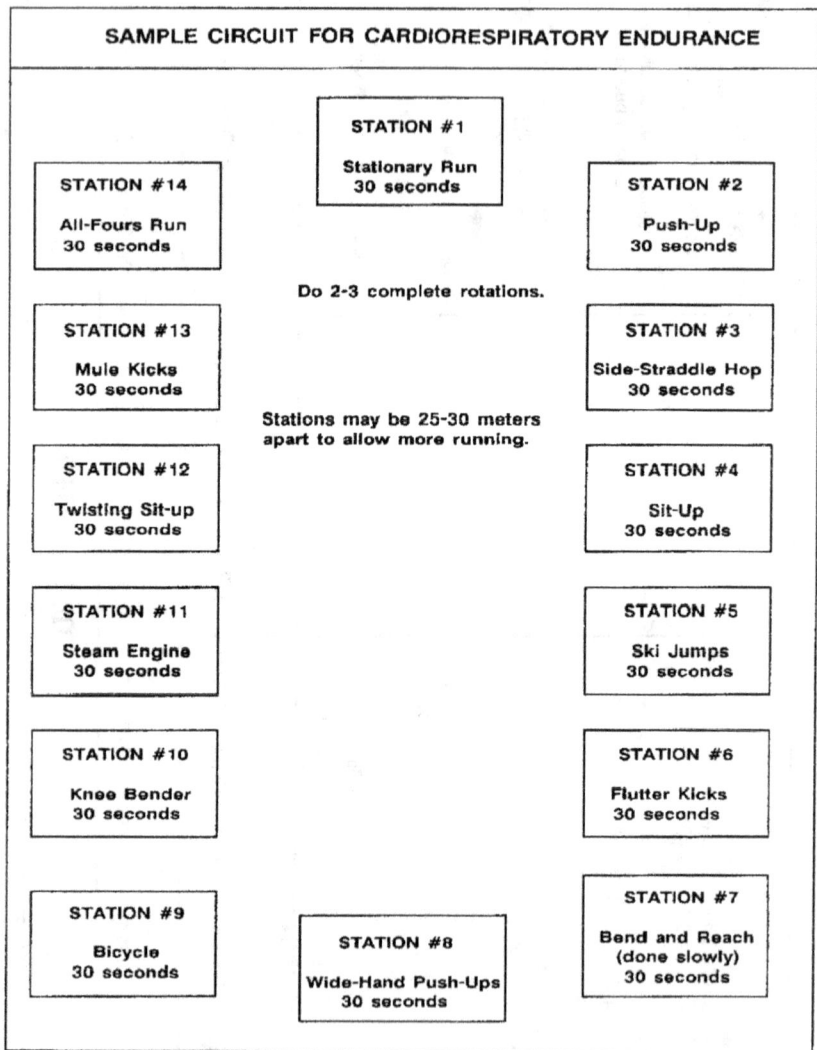

Source: FM 21-20, Physical Fitness Training, HQ Department of the Army, p. 7-4, Figure 7-1

SAMPLE CIRCUIT FOR STRENGTH DEVELOPMENT

STATION #1

Leg Press
8-12 reps

STATION #13

Incline Sit-Up
8-12 reps

STATION #2

Leg Raise
8-12 reps

Do 1-2 complete rotations.
Lift weight with slow,
controlled movements.

STATION #12

Biceps Curl
8-12 reps

STATION #3

Leg Extension
8-12 reps

Try to achieve muscle
failure within 8-12 reps.

STATION #11

Triceps Extension
8-12 reps

STATION #4

Leg Curl
8-12 reps

STATION #10

Shrug
8-12 reps

STATION #5

Heel Raise
8-12 reps

STATION #9

Lat Pull-Down
8-12 reps

STATION #6

Bench Press
8-12 reps

STATION #8

Military Press
8-12 reps

STATION #7

Seated Row
8-12 reps

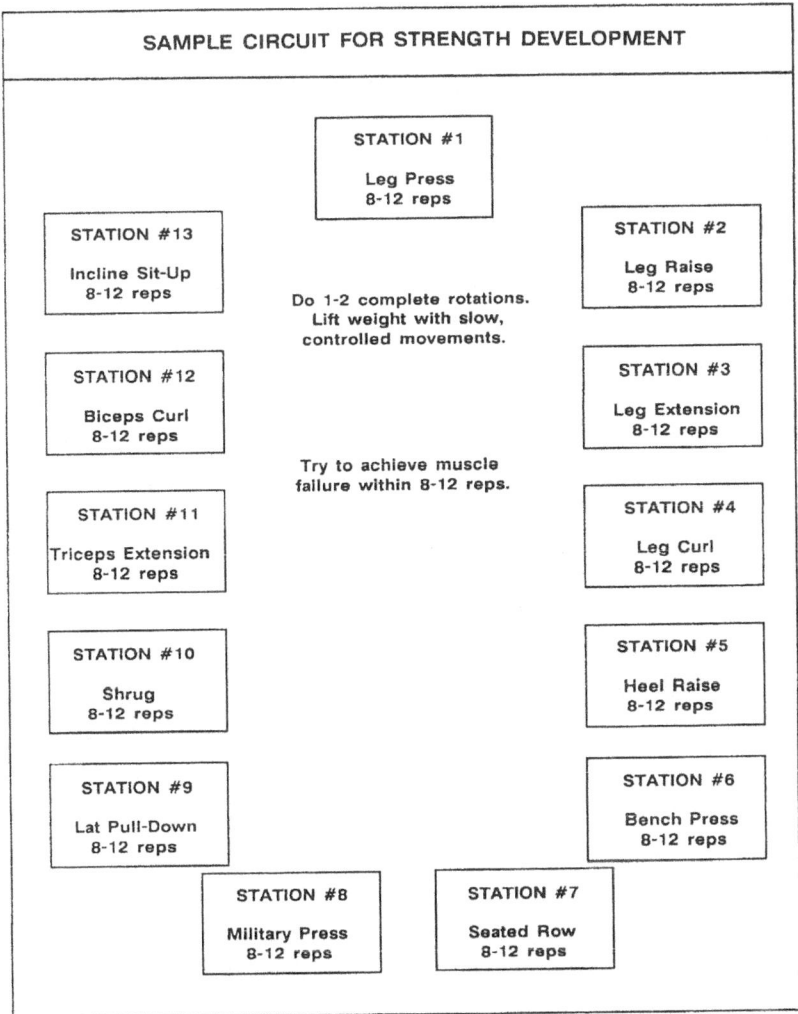

Source: FM 21-20, Physical Fitness Training, HQ Department of the Army, p. 7-4, Figure 7-1

SAMPLE CIRCUIT FOR
PUSH-UP AND SIT-UP IMPROVEMENT

STATION #1

Elevated Push-Up
30 seconds

STATION #8

Bicycle
30 seconds

STATION #2

Twisting Sit-Up
30 seconds

Do 1-2 complete rotations.

STATION #7

Close-Hand Push-Up
30 seconds

STATION #3

Parallel Dips
30 seconds

Time may decrease to 20 sec
on the second rotation.

STATION #6

Flutter Kick
30 seconds

STATION #4

Sit-Up
30 seconds

Move immediately from
station to station. If too
fatigued, push-ups may be
done on the knees.

STATION #5

Wide-Hand Push-Up
30 seconds

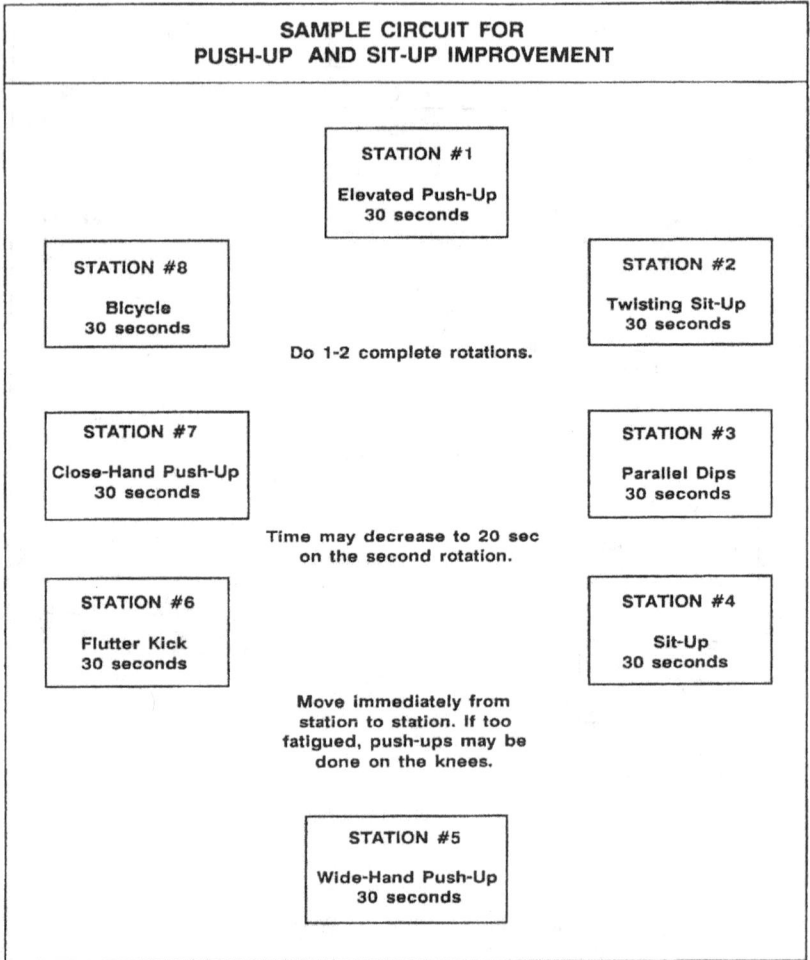

Source: FM 21-20, Physical Fitness Training, HQ Department of the Army, p. 7-4, Figure 7-1

SAMPLE PUSH-UP AND AB CIRCUITS

TIMED SETS			
SET NO.	**ACTIVITY**	**TIME PERIOD**	**REST INTERVAL**
1	Push-ups	45 seconds	0
2	Sit-ups	45 seconds	0
3	Push-ups	30 seconds	0
4	Sit-ups	30 seconds	0
5	Push-ups	30 seconds	0
6	Sit-ups	30 seconds	0

TIMED SETS			
SET NO.	**ACTIVITY**	**TIME PERIOD**	**REST INTERVAL**
1	Regular Push-ups	30 seconds	30 seconds
2	Wide-hand Push-ups	30 seconds	30 seconds
3	Close-hand Push-ups	30 seconds	30 seconds
4	Regular Push-ups	20 seconds	30 seconds
5	Regular Push-ups done on knees	30 seconds	30 seconds
6	Regular Sit-ups	60 seconds	30 seconds
7	Abdominal Twists	40 seconds	30 seconds
8	Curl-ups	30 seconds	30 seconds
9	Abdominal Crunches	30 seconds	End

Source: FM 21-20, Physical Fitness Training, HQ Department of the Army, p. 7-4, Figure 7-1

E

WORKOUT LOG

Date	Type of Exercise	Time (minutes)	Distance (miles)	Exercise Intensity	Workout Notes (ex. weather, injuries, how the session felt, etc)
				Easy Medium Hard	
				Easy Medium Hard	
				Easy Medium Hard	
				Easy Medium Hard	
				Easy Medium Hard	
				Easy Medium Hard	
				Easy Medium Hard	
				Easy Medium Hard	
				Easy Medium Hard	
				Easy Medium Hard	
				Easy Medium Hard	
				Easy Medium Hard	
				Easy Medium Hard	
				Easy Medium Hard	
				Easy Medium Hard	

F

Physical Activity Readiness Questionnaire

Also known as PAR-Q

The Physical Activity Readiness Questionnaire developed by the British Columbia Ministry of Health and the Multidisciplinary Board on Exercise (MABE). It is designed for self-screening by anyone who is planning to start an exercise programme that includes moderate to strenuous activity, such as aerobics, jogging, cycling, power walking, and swimming.

Regular physical activity is fun and healthy, and increasingly more people are starting to become more active everyday. Being more active is very safe for most people. However, some people should check with their doctor before they start becoming much more physically active.

If you are planning to become much more physically active than you are now, start by answering the seven questions in the box below. If you are between the ages of 15 and 69, the PAR-Q will tell you if you should check with your doctor before you start. If you are over 69 years of age and you are not used to being very active, check with your doctor.

Common sense is you best guide when you answer these questions. Please read the question carefully and answer each one honestly and answer with YES or NO.

PAR-Q QUESTIONS ON NEXT PAGE

Answer each question with YES or NO:

1. Has your doctor ever said that you have a heart condition and that you should only do physical activity recommended by a doctor?

2. Do you feel pain in your chest when you do physical activity?

3. In the past month, have you had chest pain when you were not doing physical activity?

4. Do you lose your balance because of dizziness or do you ever lose consciousness?

5. Do you have a bone or joint problem that could be made worse by a change in your physical activity?

6. Is your doctor currently prescribing drugs (for example, water pills) for your blood pressure or heart condition?

7. Do you know of any other reason why you should not do physical activity?

If you answered yes to one or more questions
talk with your doctor by phone or in person BEFORE you start becoming much more physically active or BEFORE you have a fitness appraisal. Tell your doctor about the PAR-Q and which questions you answered YES.

You may be able to do any activity you want - as long as you start slowly and build up gradually. Or, you may need to restrict your activities to those which are safe for you. Talk with you doctor about the kinds of activities you wish to participate in and follow his/her advice.

Find out which community programs are safe and helpful for you.

No to all questions:

If you answered NO honestly to all PAR-Q questions, you can be reasonably sure that you can:

·   Start becoming much more physically active.
    Begin slowly and build up gradually. This is the safest and easiest way to go.

·   Take part in a fitness appraisal.
    This is an excellent way to determine you basic fitness so that you can plan the best way for you to live actively.

Delay becoming much more active:

If you are not feeling well because of a temporary illness such as cold or a fever - wait until you feel better; or if you are or may be pregnant - talk to your doctor before you start becoming more active.

*Please note: If your health changes so that you then answer **YES** to any of the above questions, tell your fitness or health professional. Ask whether you should change you physical activity plan.*

Informed Use of the PAR-Q.

Lt. Col. Bob Weinstein, USAR-Ret., The Health Colonel Corporation, and their agents assume no liability for persons who undertake physical activity, and if in doubt after completing this questionnaire consult your doctor prior to physical activity.

Physical Readiness Questionnaire Revised 1994

G

MAJOR MUSCLE GROUPS

The Major Skeletal Muscles of the Human Body

Sternocleidomastoid

Rhomboids

Trapezius

Deltoids

Pectoralis Major
(Pectorals)

Triceps

Biceps

Erector Spinae

Latissimus
Dorsi

External
Obliques

Gluteals

Rectus
Abdominis
(Abdominals)

Hip Adductors

Quadriceps

Hamstrings

Gastrocnemius and
Soleus
(Calves)

Tibialis Anterior

The iliopsoas muscle (a hip flexor) cannot be seen as it lies beneath other muscles.
It attaches to the lumbar, the pelvis, the vertebrae and the femur.

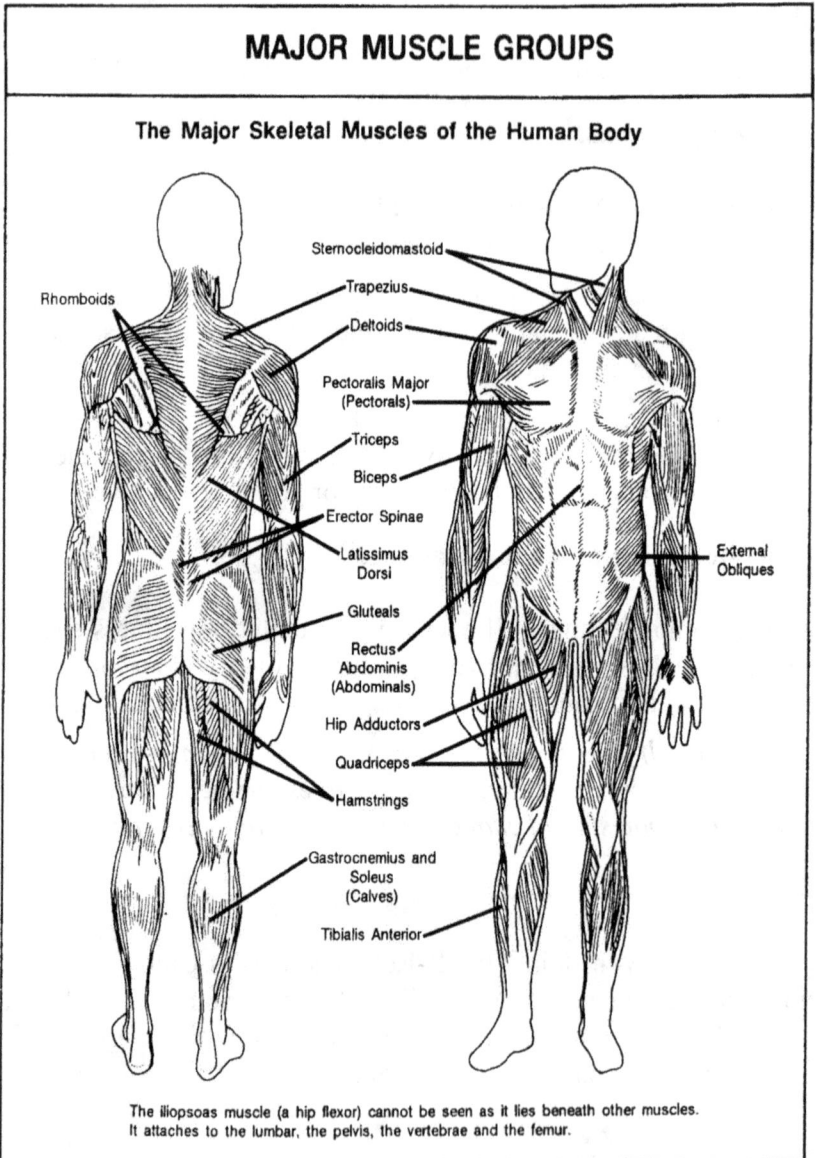

*Source: FM 21-20, Physical Fitness Training, HQ Department of the Army,
Figure 3-5*

H

MAJOR MUSCLE GROUP(S) EXERCISES

BEGINNING EXERCISE PROGRAM

NAME OF EXERCISE | **MAJOR MUSCLE GROUP(S) WORKED***

1. Leg press or squat — ---Quadriceps, Gluteals
2. Leg curl — ---Hamstrings
3. Heel raise — ---Gastrocnemius
4. Bench press — ---Pectorals, Triceps, Deltoids
5. Lat pull-down or pull-up — ---Latissimus Dorsi, Biceps
6. Overhead press — ---Deltoids, Triceps
7. Sit-up — ---Rectus Abdominus, Iliopsoas, oblique muscles
8. Bent-leg dead-lift — ---Erector Spinae, Quadriceps, Gluteals

---

MORE ADVANCED EXERCISE PROGRAM

NAME OF EXERCISE | **MAJOR MUSCLE GROUP(S) WORKED**

1. Leg press or squat — ---Quadriceps, Gluteals
2. Leg raises — ---Iliopsoas (hip flexors)
3. Leg extension — ---Quadriceps
4. Leg curl — ---Hamstrings
5. Heel raise — ---Gastrocnemius, Soleus
6. Bench press — ---Pectorals, Triceps, Deltoids
7. Seated row — ---Rhomboids, Latissimus dorsi, Biceps
8. Overhead press — ---Deltoids, Triceps
9. Lat pull-down or pull-up — ---Latissimus dorsi, Biceps
10. Shoulder shrug — ---Upper trapezius
11. Triceps extension — ---Triceps
12. Biceps curl — ---Biceps
13. Sit-up — ---Rectus abdominus, iliopsoas
14. Bent-leg dead lift — ---Erector spinae, Quadriceps, Gluteals
15. Neck flexion — ---Sternocleidomastoid
16. Neck extension — ---Upper trapezius

Source: FM 21-20, Physical Fitness Training, HQ Department of the Army, Figure 3-3 and 3-6

I

CONTRACT FOR
CHANGE OF A LIFESTYLE HABIT
"Values Determine Behavior"

1. I want to change the following lifestyle habit:

_____

_____

_____

2. I want to change this habit for the following reasons:

_____

_____

_____

_____

_____

_____

_____

3. If I changed this habit, I feel I would:

_____

_____

_____

_____

_____

_____

4. The results of the change by me:

_____

_____

_____

_____

_____

___

_____

5. I plan to make this change in the following manner (list specific steps or action plans for creating this change).

_____

_____

_____

_____

_____

6. My plan for evaluating my success will include:

_____

_____

_____

_____

_____

I agree to discuss further my change in my lifestyle habit with
_____ by

_____ (date).

I agree to discuss with _____
his/her success in changing a lifestyle habit by
_____ (date).

_____
Signature of partner

J

WEIGHT LOSS MENU 1,200
1200 Calories, Weight Loss Menu

	Energy (kcal)	Fat (GM)	% Fat	Exchange for:
Breakfast				
Whole Wheat Bread, 1 med. slice	70	1.2	15	(1 Bread/Starch)
Jelly, regular, 2 tsp	30	0	0	(½ Fruit)
Cereal, Shredded Wheat, ½ cup	104	1	4	(1 Bread/Starch)
Milk, 1%, 1 cup	102	3	23	(1 Milk)
Orange Juice ¾ cup	78	0	0	(1 ½ Fruit)
Coffee, Regular, 1 cup	5	0	0	(Free)
Breakfast Total	389	5.2	10	
Lunch				
Roast Beef Sandwich				
Whole Wheat Bread, 2 med. slice	139	2.4	15	(2 Bread/Starch)
Lean Roast Beef, unseasoned 2 oz	60	1.5	23	(2 Lean Protein)
Lettuce, 1 Leaf	1	0	0	
Tomato 3 med. slices	10	0	0	(1 Vegetable)
Mayonnaise, low-calorie, 1 tsp	15	1.7	96	(1/3 Fat)
Apple, 1 med.	80	0	0	(1 Fruit)
Water, 1 cup	0	0	0	(Free)
Lunch Total	305	56	16	
Dinner				
Salmon, 2 oz edible	103	5	40	(2 Lean Protein)
Vegetable oil, 1 ½ tsps	60	7	100	(1 ½ Fat)
Baked Potato, ¾ med.	100	0	0	(1 Bread/Starch)
Margarine, 1 tsp	34	4	100	(1 Fat)
Green Beans seasoned, with margarine, ½ cup	52	2	4	(1 Vegetable)(½ Fat)
Carrots, seasoned	35	2	0	(1 Vegetable)
White Dinner Roll, 1 sm.	70	2	26	(1 Bread/Starch)
Iced Tea, unsweetened, 1 cup	0	0	0	(Free)
Water, 2 cups	0	0	0	(Free)
Dinner Total	454	20	39	

1200 Calories, Weight Loss Menu (pg 2)

	Energy (kcal)	Fat (GM)	%Fat	Exchange for:
Snacks				
Popcorn, 2 ½ cups	69	0	0	(1 Bread/Star ch)
Margine, ¾ tsp	30	3	100	(¾ Fat)
Totals	1247	34-36	24-26	

Calories	1,247	SFA, % kcals:	7
Total Carb. %kcals	58	Cholesterol, mg.	96
Total Fat, %kcals	26	Protein, %kcals	19
Sodium, mg:	1,043		

Note: Calories have been rounded

1,200: 100% RDA met for all nutrients except Vit. E 80%, Vit. B2 96%, Vit. B6 94%, Calcium 68%, Iron 63%, Zinc 73%
   * No salt added in recipe preparation or as seasoning. Consume at lease 32 oz. Water

Source: Department of Health and Human Services, National Institute of Health, National Health, Lung and Blood Institute, Obesity Education Initiative

K

WEIGHT LOSS MENU 1,600

1600 Calories, Weight Loss Menu

	Energy (kcal)	Fat (GM)	% Fat	Exchange for:
Breakfast				
Whole Wheat Bread, 1 med. slice	70	1.2	15.4	(1 Bread/Starch)
Jelly, regular, 2 tsp	30	0	0	(½ Fruit)
Cereal, Shredded Wheat, 1 cup	207	2	8	(2 Bread/Starch)
Milk, 1%, 1 cup	102	3	23	(1 Milk)
Orange Juice ¾ cup	78	0	0	(1 ½ Fruit)
Coffee, Regular, 1 cup	5	0	0	(Free)
Milk, 1% 1 oz.	13	0.3	23	(1/8 Milk)
Breakfast Total	505	6.5	10	
Lunch				
Roast Beef Sandwich				
Whole Wheat Bread, 2 med. slice	139	2.4	15	(2 Bread/Starch)
Lean Roast Beef, unseasoned 2 oz	60	1.5	23	(2 Lean Protein)
American Cheese, low-fat and low sodium, 1 slice (¾ oz.)	46	1.8	36	(1 Lean Protein)
Lettuce, 1 Leaf	1	0	0	
Tomato 3 med. slices	10	0	0	(1 Vegetable)
Mayonnaise, low-calorie, 2 tsp	30	3.3	99	(1/3 Fat)
Apple, 1 med.	80	0	0	(1 Fruit)
Water, 1 cup	0	0	0	(Free)
Lunch Total	366	9	22	
Dinner				
Salmon, 3 oz edible	155	7	40	(3 Lean Protein)
Vegetable oil, 1 ½ tsps	60	7	100	(1 ½ Fat)
Baked Potato, ¾ med.	100	0	0	(1 Bread/Starch)
Margarine, 1 tsp	34	4	100	(1 Fat)
Green Beans seasoned, with margarine, ½ cup	52	2	4	(1 Vegetable)(½ Fat)
Carrots, seasoned w/margerine ½ cup	52	2	4	(1 Vegetable)
White Dinner Roll, 1 med.	80	3	33	(1 Bread/Starch)
Ice Milk, ½ cup	92	3	28	(½ Fat)
Iced Tea, unsweetened, 1 cup	0	0	0	(Free)
Water, 2 cups	0	0	0	(Free)
Dinner Total	625	28	38	
Snacks				
Popcorn, 2 ½ cups	69	0	0	(1 Bread/Starch)
Margine, 1 ½ tsp	58	6.5	100	(1 ½ Fat)

1600 Calories, Weight Loss Menu (pg 2)

	Energy (kcal)	Fat (GM)	%Fat	Exchange for:
Totals	1613	50	28	

Calories	1,613	SFA, % kcals:	8
Total Carb. %kcals	55	Cholesterol, mg.	142
Total Fat, %kcals	29	Protein, %kcals	19
Sodium, mg:	1,341		

Note: Calories have been rounded

1,600: 100% RDA met for all nutrients except Vit. E 99%, Iron 73%, Zinc 91%
* No salt added in recipe preparation or as seasoning. Consume at lease 32 oz. Water

A 5'4", 175 lb woman and a 5'8", 200 lb man (both with a BMI of 30) would have energy expenditures of approximately 2,500 calorie and 3,000 calories/day respectively (15 calories per pound). However, the underreporting of caloric intake has been estimated to be in the range of 400 to 900 calories per day. Thus, a 1600 calorie per day diet should yield a deficit of about 500 to 1000 calories per day, or 1 to 2 pounds per week weight loss. If you lose 4 lbs in 1 month, you are losing about 500 calories per day or 1 lb per week. Both total amount of weight lost as well as weight maintenance may be improved by increasing the number of minutes of activities of daily living, chores and exercise.

Source: Department of Health and Human Services, National Institute of Health, National Health, Lung and Blood Institute, Obesity Education Initiative

L

FOOD DIARY

HOW MUCH DO YOU EAT?

Did you know that there's a difference between servings and helpings?

Serving: A serving is a measured amount of food, like 1/2 cup or one ounce. It's like a measuring tool.

Helping: A helping is what most people usually eat. Helpings may be larger or smaller than servings. It all depends on how much you eat.

Pyramid Serving: A Pyramid serving may be a smaller amount of food than what you usually eat. A good way to help you figure out what you should be eating is to keep a Food Diary. It will show you where you need to fill in some of your Food Guide Pyramid gaps.

Photocopy the food diary and use it to make notes on what you eat today - make extra copies for other days - refer to them so you can improve on how you eat.

Source: Nutrition.gov. Nutrition.gov provides easy access to the best food and nutrition information from across the federal government. It serves as a gateway to reliable information on nutrition, healthy eating, physical activity, and food safety for consumers.

FOOD DIARY

Time	Types of Foods	Helpings of Food	Pyramid Serving Size
Breakfast			
Lunch			
Dinner			
Snacks			

FITT Factors Applied to Conditioning Programs for Muscular Endurance and/or Strength		
Muscular Strength	Muscular Endurance	Muscular Strength and Muscular Endurance
3 times/week	3-5 times/week	3 times/week
3-7 RM*	12+ RM	8-12 RM
The time required to do 3-7 repetitions of each resistance exercise	The time required to do 12+ repetitions of each resistance exercise	The time required to do 8-12 repetitions of each resistance exercise
Free Weights Resistance Machines Partner-Resisted Exercises Body-Weight Exercises (Push-ups/Sit-ups/Pull-ups/Dips, etc.) * RM = Repetition Maximum		

Source: FM 21-20, Physical Fitness Training, US Department of the Army, p. 3-3, 30 September 1992

M

SERVING SIZE CARD FOR WALLET

SERVING SIZE CARD:
Cut out and fold on the dotted line. Laminate for longtime use.

---

1 Serving Looks Like . . .

GRAIN PRODUCTS

1 cup of cereal flakes = fist

1 pancake = compact disc

½ cup of cooked rice, pasta, or potato = ½ baseball

1 slice of bread = cassette tape

1 piece of cornbread = bar of soap

---

1 Serving Looks Like . . .

VEGETABLES AND FRUIT

1 cup of salad greens = baseball

1 baked potato = fist

1 med. fruit = baseball

½ cup of fresh fruit = ½ baseball

¼ cup of raisins = large egg

---

1 Serving Looks Like . . .

DAIRY AND CHEESE

1½ oz. cheese = 4 stacked dice or 2 cheese slices

½ cup of ice cream = ½ baseball

FATS

1 tsp. margarine or spreads = 1 dice

---

1 Serving Looks Like . . .

MEAT AND ALTERNATIVES

3 oz. meat, fish, and poultry = deck of cards

3 oz. grilled/baked fish = checkbook

2 Tbsp. peanut butter = ping pong ball

Source: US Nat'l Heart Lung and Blood Institute

N

Calories Burned: Exercise and Food Charts
Beverages

	Smoothie, Ban. Berry, 16 oz	Caramel Frappucino, 16 oz.	Red wine, 5 oz	Beer, 12 oz.	Orange Juice, 12 oz.	Soft drink, 12 oz.
	Jamba Juice	Starbucks	Generic	Generic	Generic	Generic
	518 cal.	**380 cal.**	**125 cal.**	**278 cal.**	**140 cal.**	**150 cal.**
Aerobics Active	65 min	48 min	16 min	35 min	18 min	19 min
Walking 3 mph	95 min	70 min	23 min	51 min	26 min	28 min
Jogging 5 mph	65 min	48 min	16 min	35 min	18 min	19 min
Biking Leisure	115 min	85 min	28 min	62 min	31 min	34 min
Dancing Energetic	80 min	59 min	20 min	43 min	22 min	23 min

Breads & Pastries

	Bagel plain	White Bread, slice	Croissant, plain	Dinner Roll	Muffin Blueberry	Scone, Blueberry
	Einstein's	Generic	Starbucks	Generic	Einstein's	Starbucks
	260 cal.	**80 cal.**	**440 cal.**	**87 cal.**	**480 cal.**	**460 cal.**
Aerobics Active	33 min	10 min	55 min	11 min	60 min	58 min
Walking 3 mph	47 min	70 min	80 min	16 min	87 min	84 min
Jogging 5 mph	33 min	10 min	55 min	11 min	60 min	58 min
Biking Leisure	58 min	18 min	98 min	20 min	107 min	102 min
Dancing Energetic	40 min	12 min	68 min	14 min	74 min	71 min

Calories Burned: Exercise and Food Charts

Fast Food

	Pizza Slice 3.6 oz cheese	Big Mac	French Fries large	Spagetti w/ Meat Balls 18.9 oz.	Turkey Breast Wrap	5 Chicken Wings
	Generic	McDonald's	McDonald's	Pizza Hut	Subway	Hooters
	272 cal.	540 cal.	500 cal.	850 cal.	270 cal.	866 cal.
Aerobics Active	35 min	70 min	65 min	107 min	35 min	110 min
Walking 3 mph	55 min	100 min	90 min	155 min	50 min	160 min
Jogging 5 mph	35 min	70 min	65 min	107 min	35 min	110 min
Biking Leisure	60 min	120 min	115 min	190 min	60 min	200 min
Dancing Energetic	45 min	85 min	80 min	130 min	40 min	135 min

Fruit

	Apple medium	Banana medium	Raisens 4 oz	Strawberries 4 oz	Orange medium	Blueberries 4 oz
	72 cal.	105 cal.	340 cal.	36 cal.	64 cal.	45 cal.
Aerobics Active	9 min	13 min	43 min	5 min	8 min	5 min
Walking 3 mph	13 min	19 min	62 min	7 min	12 min	8 min
Jogging 5 mph	9 min	13 min	43 min	5 min	8 min	5 min
Biking Leisure	16 min	23 min	75 min	8 min	14 min	10 min
Dancing Energetic	11 min	16 min	52 min	6 min	10 min	7 min

Calories Burned: Exercise and Food Charts

Vegetables

	White Potato medium	Carrots Cup, grated	Peas cup	String beans cup	Spinach cup	Sweet Potato medium
	164 cal.	**52 cal.**	**117 cal.**	**34 cal.**	**7 cal.**	**103 cal.**
Aerobics Active	20 min	7 min	15 min	4 min	1 min	13 min
Walking 3 mph	30 min	10 min	21 min	5 min	1 min	13 min
Jogging 5 mph	20 min	7 min	15 min	4 min	1 min	13 min
Biking Leisure	36 min	12 min	26 min	8 min	2 min	23 min
Dancing Energetic	25 min	8 min	18 min	5 min	1 min	16 min

Nuts, Beans and Rice

	Almonds Dry roasted cup	Walnuts Cup, chopped	Peanuts Dry roasted cup	Black beans cup	White Rice cup	Brown Rice cup
	546 cal.	**785 cal.**	**854 cal.**	**280 cal.**	**242 cal.**	**218 cal.**
Aerobics Active	68 min	98 min	107 min	35 min	30 min	27 min
Walking 3 mph	99 min	143 min	155 min	51 min	44 min	40 min
Jogging 5 mph	68 min	98 min	107 min	35 min	30 min	27 min
Biking Leisure	121 min	174 min	190 min	62 min	54 min	48 min
Dancing Energetic	84 min	121 min	131 min	43 min	37 min	33 min

O

List of Calories in Foods

Food	Serving Size	Calories
Bacon	2 slices	80
Brownie	2 inch square	243
Caesar salad	10 oz w/dressg	520
Carrot, fresh	One medium	35
Cheesecake	¼ of 19 oz cake	330
Chicken breast	6 oz	280
Coffee w/sugar	Cup+2 tsp sgr	32
Egg white	Large	17
Egg with yoke	Large	78
Milk	8 oz	160
Oatmeal	Cup cooked	147
Oatmeal cookie	113gr. Einsteins	600
Orange	180 gr.	85
Orange Juice	8 oz	112
Pancakes	2 cakes, 200gr.	450
Pasta	2 cups cooked	600
Potato chips	1 oz	150
Potato, baked	7 oz	200
Swiss Cheese	One slice	70
Tortilla chips	4 oz	200
Tuna fish	4.5 oz	120
Watermelon	Cup diced	46
White bread	1 slice	67
Yogurt, fruit	8 oz	120

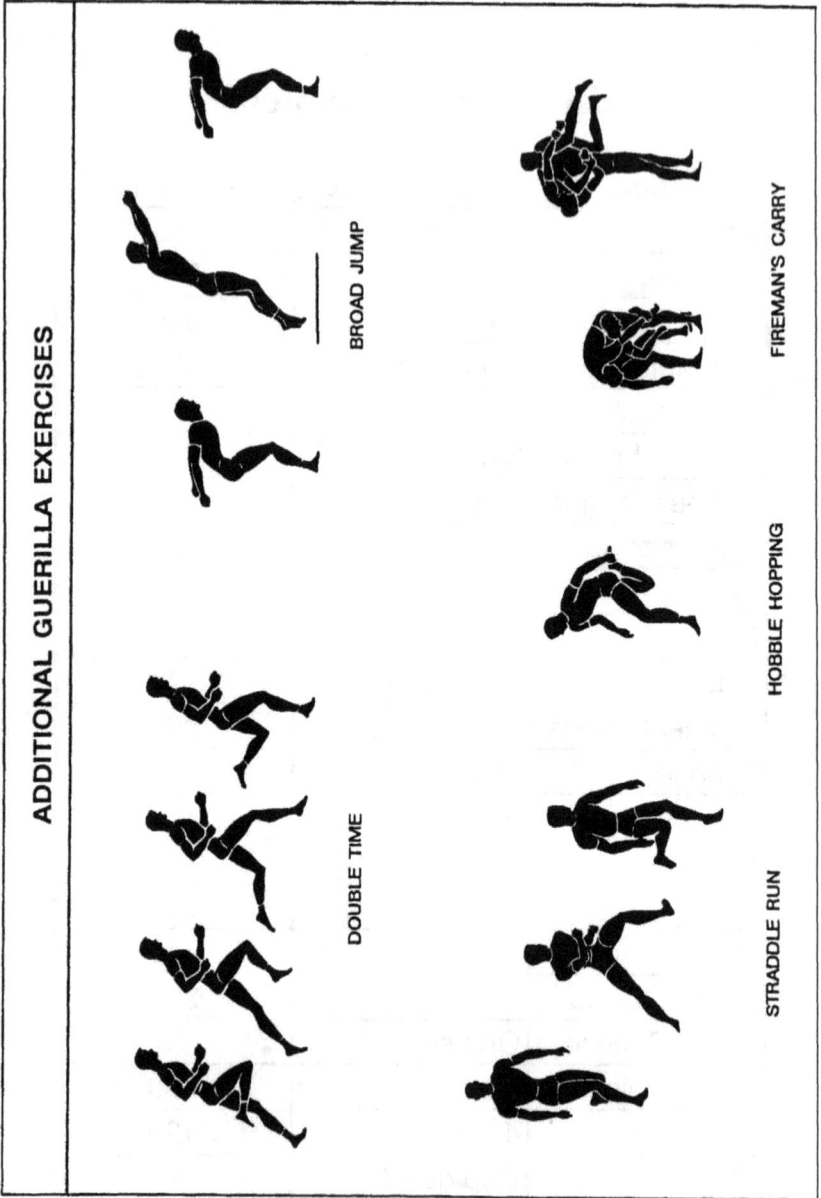

Source: FM 21-20, Physical Fitness Training, US Department of the Army, p. 7-26, 30 September 1992

P

MYPYRAMID FOOD AND CALORIE NEEDS CHARTS

MyPyramid

Food Intake Patterns

The suggested amounts of food to consume from the basic food groups, subgroups, and oils to meet recommended nutrient intakes at 12 different calorie levels.

Nutrient and energy contributions from each group are calculated according to the nutrient-dense forms of foods in each group (e.g., lean meats and fat-free milk).

The table also shows the discretionary calorie allowance that can be accommodated within each calorie level, in addition to the suggested amounts of nutrient-dense forms of foods in each group.

Source: US Department of Agriculture, Center for Nutrition Policy and Promotion, April 2005

DAILY AMOUNT OF FOOD FROM EACH GROUP

My Pyramid 2

Daily Amount of Food From Each Group
See footnotes 1-8 on next page

Calorie Level[1]	1,000	1,200	1,400	1,600	1,800	2,000	2,200	2,400	2,600	2,800	3,000	3,200
Fruits[2]	1 cup	1 cup	1.5 cups	1.5 cups	1.5 cups	2 cups	2 cups	2 cups	2 cups	2.5 cups	2.5 cups	2.5 cups
Vegetables[3]	1 cup	1.5 cups	1.5 cups	2 cups	2.5 cups	2.5 cups	3 cups	3 cups	3.5 cups	3.5 cups	4 cups	4 cups
Grains[4]	3 oz-eq	4 oz-eq	5 oz-eq	5 oz-eq	6 oz-eq	6 oz-eq	7 oz-eq	8 oz-eq	9 oz-eq	10 oz-eq	10 oz-eq	10 oz-eq
Meat and Beans[5]	2 oz-eq	3 oz-eq	4 oz-eq	5 oz-eq	5 oz-eq	5.5 oz-eq	6 oz-eq	6.5 oz-eq	6.5 oz-eq	7 oz-eq	7 oz-eq	7 oz-eq
Milk[6]	2 cups	2 cups	2 cups	3 cups	3 cups	3 cups	3 cups	3 cups	3 cups	3 cups	3 cups	3 cups
Oils[7]	3 tsp	4 tsp	4 tsp	5 tsp	5 tsp	6 tsp	6 tsp	7 tsp	8 tsp	8 tsp	10 tsp	11 tsp
Discretionary calorie allowance[8]	165	171	171	132	195	267	290	362	410	426	512	648

Source: US Department of Agriculture, Center for Nutrition Policy and Promotion, April 2005

FOOTNOTES FOR TABLE DAILY AMOUNT OF FOOD

Footnotes for table Daily Amount of Food from Each Group:

1 Calorie Levels are set across a wide range to accommodate the needs of different individuals. The attached table "Estimated Daily Calorie Needs" can be used to help assign individuals to the food intake pattern at a particular calorie level.

2 Fruit Group includes all fresh, frozen, canned, and dried fruits and fruit juices. In general, 1 cup of fruit or 100% fruit juice, or 1/2 cup of dried fruit can be considered as 1 cup from the fruit group.

3 Vegetable Group includes all fresh, frozen, canned, and dried vegetables and vegetable juices. In general, 1 cup of raw or cooked vegetables or vegetable juice, or 2 cups of raw leafy greens can be considered as 1 cup from the vegetable group.

4 Grains Group includes all foods made from wheat, rice, oats, cornmeal, barley, such as bread, pasta, oatmeal, breakfast cereals, tortillas, and grits. In general, 1 slice of bread, 1 cup of ready-to-eat cereal, or 1/2 cup of cooked rice, pasta, or cooked cereal can be considered as 1 ounce equivalent from the grains group. At least half of all grains consumed should be whole grains.

5 Meat & Beans Group in general, 1 ounce of lean meat, poultry, or fish, 1 egg, 1 Tbsp. peanut butter, 1/4 cup cooked dry beans, or 1/2 ounce of nuts or seeds can be considered as 1 ounce equivalent from the meat and beans group.

6 Milk Group includes all fluid milk products and foods made from milk that retain their calcium content, such as yogurt and cheese. Foods made from milk that have little to no calcium, such as cream cheese, cream, and butter, are not part of the group. Most milk group choices should be fat-free or low-fat. In general, 1 cup of milk or yogurt, 1 1/2 ounces of natural cheese, or 2 ounces of processed cheese can be considered as 1 cup from the milk group.

7 Oils include fats from many different plants and from fish that are liquid at room temperature, such as canola, corn, olive, soybean, and sunflower oil. Some foods are naturally high in oils, like nuts, olives, some fish, and avocados. Foods that are mainly oil include mayonnaise, certain salad dressings, and soft margarine.

8 Discretionary Calorie Allowance is the remaining amount of calories in a food intake pattern after accounting for the calories needed for all food groups—using forms of foods that are fat-free or low-fat and with no added sugars.

Source: US Department of Agriculture, Center for Nutrition Policy and Promotion, April 2005

ESTIMATED DAILY CALORIE NEEDS

Source: US Department of Agriculture, Center for Nutrition Policy and Promotion, April 2005

To determine which food intake pattern to use for an individual, the following chart gives an estimate of individual calorie needs. The calorie range for each age/sex group is based on physical activity level, from sedentary to active.

		Calorie Range	
		Sedentary →	Active →
Children			
	2–3 years	1,000	1,400
Females			
	4–8 years	1,200	1,800
	9–13	1,600	2,200
	14–18	1,800	2,400
	19–30	2,000	2,400
	31–50	1,800	2,200
	51+	1,600	2,200
Males			
	4–8 years	1,400	2,000
	9–13	1,800	2,600
	14–18	2,200	3,200
	19–30	2,400	3,000
	31–50	2,200	3,000
	51+	2,000	2,800

Sedentary means a lifestyle that includes only the light physical activity associated with typical day-to-day life.

Active means a lifestyle that includes physical activity equivalent to walking more than 3 miles per day at 3 to 4 miles per hour, in addition to

Q

FREE RESOURCES
ON EXERCISE AND HEALTHY EATING

Health, Nutrition and Exercise
www.hhs.gov
US Dept of Health and Human Services

Exercise Activity for Everyone
US National Library of Medicine and National Institute of Health
www.nlm.nih.gov/medlineplus

Exercise for Older Adults
US Dept. of Health and Human Services
www.nihseniorhealth.gov

Dietary Guidelines for Americans
US Dept. of Agriculture
www.cnpp.usda.gov
www.mypyramid.gov

Free BMI Calculators
The President's Challenge
President's Council on Physical Fitness and Sports
www.presidentschallenge.org
www.nhlbisupport.com/bmi/
www.fitness.gov

Look up Calories or Nutrients in Food
www.nal.usda.gov/fnic/foodcomp/search

Youth Weight Management
www.nutrition.gov

Menu Planner
National Heart, Lung and Blood Institute
http://hp2010.nhlbihin.net/menuplanner/menu.cgi

Index

C

D

E

I

J

K

L

S

Y

More Products from the Health Colonel
Use quick order form on next page or go to
www.The HealthColonel.com for EASY ONLINE ORDERING.

Get Your Priorities Straight

Put an end to indecisiveness and take back control of your life.
Learn to move out with confidence and purpose. Learn to overcome
life obstacles. Discover your true life priorities and how to imple-
ment them. Find out how to reinvent your life into the true you that
is already inside and waiting to be allowed to live life to the fullest.
Discover the ultimate law of happiness and learn how to apply it
today.
Audio CD: $11.95 (30 min.)

Quotes to Live By

My personal journey to seek out wisdom and improvement in my
life and the lives of others has resulted in this collection of quotes.
May they inspire you or someone you know to be a better person
and always take the high road when faced with challenging deci-
sions. The journey is still in progress for me and will last a lifetime.
Paperback: $7.99

Six Keys to Permanent Weight-loss

Join the Fitness and Beach Boot Camp Instructor, Lt. Col. Bob
Weinstein, USAR, (ret.), on his over 60 minute journey to successful
and permanent weight loss, delivered with enthusiasm, humor and
high energy. You will tap into the vast experience of the Health
Colonel. You will talk, think and eat yourself lean after following
Colonel Weinstein's straightforward, no-nonsense, Six Keys to Per-
manent Weight Loss.
Audio CD: $11.99 (60 min.)

Change Made Easy - Your Basic Training Orders to Excellent Physical and Mental Health

Put on your commander's hat. You are about to take charge of your health. This book is a health and fitness blueprint to get America back in shape, keep Americans from dying of ill health and keep Americans strong. A combination of self-help, right eating, exercising, how to start a fitness boot camp, weight loss as well as guidance on how to lead a values-based life to the benefit of others and our society. Lots of exercise photos.
Paperback: $14.99

Eight Secrets to Longevity, Health and Fitness

An exciting journey to empower and educate you to take charge of your health and eating habits. Put on your commander's hat and take charge of your all those body parts that may not be firm as they used to. Delivered with enthusiasm, humor and high energy. You will tap into the vast experience of the Health Colonel. A Straight-forward, no-nonsense, back-to-basics approach to exercise and eating.
Audio CD: $11.99 (54 min.)

Beach Boot Camp Upper Body Blast

Suitable for all fitness levels and excellent for group exercise instruction. This video is much more than those follow-along workout routines on the market. It includes great workout tips, humor, great beach scenes and inspirational and motivational guidance all wrapped into this dynamic 29 minute program. The workout is filmed on Fort Lauderdale Beach in Florida. Join him with his group class as he equips and empowers you to take your workout to the next level. Both natural body weight exercises as well as some using an inexpensive rubber resistance band are demonstrated.
DVD Video: $14.95 (29 min.)

COMMANDER'S CHECKLIST FOR NUTRITION

PRINCIPLES OF NUTRITION

1. Eat a variety of foods.
No single food item provides all essential nutrients.

2. Maintain a desirable body weight.
Excess body fat detracts from fitness. Weight loss is achieved by increasing physical activity and decreasing total food intake, especially fats, refined sugars, and alcohol.

3. Avoid excess dietary fat.
Too much fat (especially cholesterol and saturated fat) can lead to heart disease and weight problems. Fats contain twice as many calories as equal amounts of carbohydrates or protein.

4. Avoid too much sugar.
Sweets are empty calories and may lead to dental cavities and weight problems.

5. Eat foods with adequate starch and fiber.
Eating complex carbohydrates adds to the diet and reduces symptoms of constipation.

6. Avoid too much sodium.
Eating highly-salted foods may lead to excessive sodium intake. This may be a problem for those "at risk" for high blood pressure.

7. If you drink alcoholic beverages, do so in moderation.
Alcoholic beverages are high in calories and and low in nutrients. One or two standard-size drinks daily appears to cause no harm in normal, healthy, nonpregnant adults.

8. Know the nutrition principles.
Educating soldiers maximizes efforts to improve nutritional fitness.

SUPPORTING ACTIONS

In the dining facility:
● Ensure menus provide foods from the basic 4 food groups: fruits and vegetables, meats, dairy products, and breads and cereals.
● Establish serving lines in the following order, if possible:
(1) salads, (2) fruits, (3) entrees, (4) hot vegetables, (5) breads, (6) beverages, (7) desserts.

In the dining facility, provide:
● Low-calorie menu, including short-order items at each meal. Use the Master Menu (SB 10-260) menu patterns.
● Reduced-portion sizes.
● No-calorie beverages.
● Low-calorie salad dressings.
● Posted list of caloric values of menu items, before or on the serving line.

In the dining facility, provide:
● Non-fried eggs as an alternative.
● Margarine as a butter alternative.
● Two percent milk as the primary milk in bulk dispensers.
● Skim milk in 1/2-pint cartons.
● Sauces, gravies, and margarine separately from the entree or vegetable.
● Avoid animal fats, palm oil, and hydrogenated vegetable oil.

In the dining facility, provide:
● Fruit as a dessert alternative.
● Unsweetened juices.
● No-calorie, unsweetened beverages.
● Non-nutritive, sugar substitute as a granulated sugar alternative.
● Unsweetened cereal.

In the dining facility, provide:
● Whole-grain breads, cereals and legumes.
● Fresh fruit.
● Salad bars at lunch and dinner.

● Reduce salt in recipes by 25 percent.

● Avoid alcohol; it is detrimental to good health and weight management.

● Display educational materials on nutrition; (posters, table tents, bulletin boards, and handouts).
● Provide food-service personnel with training programs on nutrition standards.
● Provide unit-training programs on nutrition for soldiers. (Use installation dietitian).

Reference: AR 30-1, Appendix J.

Source: FM 21-20, Physical Fitness Training, US Department of the Army, p. 6-4, 30 September 1992

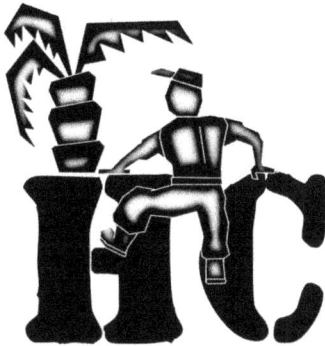

THEHEALTHCOLONEL.COM

Changing the way people think about health.

QUICK ORDER FORM

Fax orders: 866-481-2804. Send this form.

Telephone orders: Call 888-768-9892 toll-free

Email orders: thehealthcolonel@beachbootcamp.net

Postal orders: The Health Colonel, Lt. Col. Bob Weinstein, USAR-Ret., 757 SE 17th Street, #267, Fort Lauderdale, FL 33316, Telephone 954-636-5351

Please send the following books, audio CDs, DVDs:

Please send more FREE information on:

❑ Other books   ❑ Speaking/seminars

❑ Fitness Boot Camp ❑ Mailing Lists

Name:

Address:

City: State: Zip:

Telephone:

Email address:

Sales tax: Please add Florida sales tax for products shipped to Florida addresses.

Shipping:
U.S.: $4.50 for first book, CD or DVD and $2.50 for each additional product.
International: $9.50 for first product; $5.50 for each additional product (estimate).

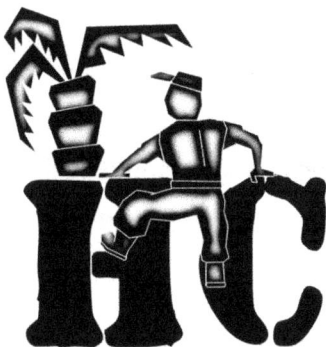

THEHEALTHCOLONEL.COM

Changing the way people think about health.

QUICK ORDER FORM

Fax orders: 866-481-2804. Send this form.

Telephone orders: Call 888-768-9892 toll-free

Email orders: thehealthcolonel@beachbootcamp.net

Postal orders: The Health Colonel, Lt. Col. Bob Weinstein, USAR-Ret., 757 SE 17th Street, #267, Fort Lauderdale, FL 33316, Telephone 954-636-5351

Please send the following books, audio CDs, DVDs:

Please send more FREE information on:

❑ Other books   ❑ Speaking/seminars

❑ Fitness Boot Camp ❑ Mailing Lists

Name:

Address:

City: State: Zip:

Telephone:

Email address:

Sales tax: Please add Florida sales tax for products shipped to Florida addresses.

Shipping:
U.S.: $4.50 for first book, CD or DVD and $2.50 for each additional product.
International: $9.50 for first product; $5.50 for each additional product (estimate).

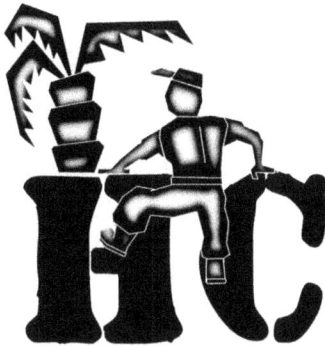

THEHEALTHCOLONEL.COM

CHANGING THE WAY PEOPLE THINK ABOUT HEALTH.

QUICK ORDER FORM

Fax orders: 866-481-2804. Send this form.

Telephone orders: Call 888-768-9892 toll-free

Email orders: thehealthcolonel@beachbootcamp.net

Postal orders: The Health Colonel, Lt. Col. Bob Weinstein, USAR-Ret., 757 SE 17th Street, #267, Fort Lauderdale, FL 33316, Telephone 954-636-5351

Please send the following books, audio CDs, DVDs:

Please send more FREE information on:

❑ Other books   ❑ Speaking/seminars

❑ Fitness Boot Camp ❑ Mailing Lists

Name:

Address:

City: State: Zip:

Telephone:

Email address:

Sales tax: Please add Florida sales tax for products shipped to Florida addresses.

Shipping:
U.S.: $4.50 for first book, CD or DVD and $2.50 for each additional product.
International: $9.50 for first product; $5.50 for each additional product (estimate).